Aspergillus & penicill...... .... the
humidity in
need a ↓ .This

✱ Dehumidifier running at all
    times in Basement

✱ HEPA Filters in Cold Weather

Antioxidants
Probotics
Brown Seaweed Detoxification
    Supplements Called
" Limu moui "

(Stacy botrys)
(Chaetomium)
(Black Mold)

Surviving Toxic Black Mold Syndrome

Mary E. Ray M.S., D.O.

Natural Health Doc LLC
St. Augustine, Florida

ISBN: 978-0692110744
Published by Natural Health Doc LLC
www.natural-health-doc.com
St. Augustine, Florida

Printed in the United States of America

To the Holy Spirit for His Guidance.

ACKNOWLEDGEMENTS:

Much thanks to my husband, John, and our two-year-old son, Sam, who have both been very patient and supportive throughout this endeavor.

Special thanks to Richard C. Short, my father, the English professor, for his help in editing; Theresa Short, my mom, for her constant moral support; Ruth Ray, my mother-in-law, for her uplifting spirit and moral support; Ginny Ray, my sister-in-law, for her uplifting spirit and words of encouragement; Lynn Beals-Becker, D.O., for her belief in me and her assistance in helping me find the cause of my health problems; Ritchie Shoemaker, M.D., for his book *Mold Warriors*; and Sandra Beals, for her support.

Thank you to Janet Schester, Jennifer Roode, Carolyn DiCuccio, Mercedes Webster D.O., June and Gordon Lawhead, Frank and Connie Frontiera, Ed Short, Mark Rojek, Kimya Nguyen D.O., Amy Kelleher, Therese Quinn, and John Ohanesian, for all their support and encouraging words.

"Don't judge any man until you have walked two moons in his moccasins."
—Native American Proverb

Table of Contents

Chapter 1
My Story

It was a crisp fall day that weekend. I had just put my ten-month-old baby boy, Sam, down for a nap. Now was my time to spring into action and get some things done around the house without interruption! I decided to start by raking leaves outside the front door. I worked for about fifteen minutes before I started to feel lightheaded. This was unusual for me, for I considered myself to be in fairly good shape. I stopped, went inside and sat down to wait for the feeling to pass. It did not. It got worse and I soon felt as though I was going to pass out. My heart was racing, my legs felt weak and I had a strange feeling of dread. I told my husband that I thought I was going to pass out and asked him to check my blood pressure and listen to my heart. My blood pressure was okay and my heart rate was 120. My husband suggested I was having a panic attack. But I hadn't been upset about anything. I had been having a nice relaxing day. It took about a half-hour for the panic attack to pass, and I eventually went to sleep.

I continued to have these panic attacks without cause at any time of day and any place. They would hit without warning and each panic attack made me more fearful of the next. Would I actually pass out during one of these attacks? That was my big fear. When driving, I was afraid to pass out behind the wheel with my ten-month-old in the back seat. If I was alone at home with my baby and passed out, what would happen to the baby? It was pure hell.

I got out my medical books and searched the Internet. The best help I got was from websites on panic attacks where I learned that the feeling of passing out is one of the symptoms some people get with panic attacks. So, if this was an anxiety disorder, did I just now suddenly develop it? I was ten months postpartum. Could this be postpartum depression? I did not feel depressed at all—I just felt anxious. So, okay, I guess it could be the anxiety component of the depression that I was feeling. Also, my son was weaning off breast-feeding, and it could be a hormonal change. But I could not find any information on weaning a child as a cause of panic attacks. My thought was that it was not something emotional but something physical.

I did not have anything to be depressed about. I had a great husband, a wonderful baby boy, a nice house on a lake, and a comfortable job. And better yet, at the end of October we had just moved our office to a new building from an older moldy building. So, we were all hoping the new office would be a healthier environment to work in. And it was a beautiful, newly remodeled, office space in a large mirrored glass building. It was much more professional than the last place that we had been working in and we were so glad to leave. The only thing I would miss about the old building was being able to open the windows.

I decided to take Xanax when I got the panic attacks. The problem was it would take a half-hour for the Xanax to work, and by then the panic attack would be almost over. But since the levels persisted awhile in the system, it would lessen any subsequent attacks.

I had seen an ear, nose and throat doctor in early November for pulsatile tinnitus (I felt my pulse in my ear) that I had since my pregnancy. He ordered an MRI to rule out aneurysms. This occurred before the panic attacks had started. I did notice at this doctor's office feeling unusually nervous and not being able to get a hold of myself and control the feeling like I normally would.

I scheduled the MRI for Dec 21. About one week before the MRI, I suddenly developed tremors, numbness in my left leg, visual impairment that was almost double vision and difficulty walking. My walking was a shuffling gait with small steps and the muscles on the insides of my thighs felt weak. My whole body was trembling inwardly—I was terrified. Thoughts of brain tumors and multiple sclerosis raced through my head. I did not know what was hitting me. I prayed to God, "Please don't let this be happening to me." I had a husband and a new baby. Why was this happening to me now?

My MRI came back showing nonspecific signs, suggestive of early demyleination. However, the neurologists (I saw two) and the radiologist friend of mine did not think it was typical of multiple sclerosis (MS). The MRI findings were nonspecific, they all said. And the symptoms and physical exam were not characteristic of MS according to both neurologists. One neurologist implied that I was crazy and the other one handed me a prescription for an antidepressant.

So, over the next seven months I would have flare-ups of the neurological symptoms, episodes of panic attacks, anxiety, vertigo, difficulty thinking clearly like my brain was not working, balance problems, abdominal pains, tremors, numbness and tingling in my legs, a weird buzzing sensation in my head, fatigue, burning muscle pains in my thighs, shooting sharp ice pick-like pains anywhere and at any time, low back pain, headaches, flu-like symptoms, a constant fever of 99 F and excessive menstrual bleeding.

I drove my poor husband crazy with a different symptom every week, but never a day without symptoms.

I am a physician and was trying to diagnose myself, since I knew something was wrong and the doctors I had seen could not give me an answer. I went through thinking I had MS, cancer, gallbladder disease, stomach ulcers, endometriosis, fibromyalgia, intestinal candidiasis, mitral valve prolapse syndrome, postpartum depression, Lyme disease and chronic fatigue syndrome. I took many different combinations of supplements depending on what symptoms were surfacing and what disease I had that week. I switched from a high protein diet to the Swanck low saturated fat, high oil and no dairy diet to a no wheat diet to a raw vegan diet and finally to the anti-candida diet with no fruit or bread or sugar. The anti-candida diet worked the best to control the symptoms but did not completely eliminate the symptoms. I was frantically jumping from one diet, supplement program and diagnosis to another diet, supplement program and diagnosis. I really don't blame my husband for thinking I had gone mad.

In my prayers I would always ask God to please point me in the right direction to find the answer. In September of 2006, almost one year later, that prayer was answered. After doing some research on the Internet, I came across some information on fungus being the cause of some illnesses. It was actually a website a patient of mine had told me about called knowthecause.com, featuring the work of Doug Kaufman Ph.D. and David Holland M.D. They both have successfully cleared up many medical conditions in patients by treating them for fungal infections. It was here that I learned about fungal mycotoxin poisoning and the symptoms it can cause. Some of the symptoms such as tremors, abdominal pain and neurological symptoms caught my eye because they matched up with some of the symptoms I had been experiencing. I learned that mycotoxins can be found in foods but that they can also come from mold in the environment. Bingo. It was then I decided to check my house for mold. Then later that same week, a physician friend of mine, Lynn Beals-Becker D.O., who had been one of the few people who did not think I had gone mad, called me and said, "Mary, I am reading a book about you and the symptoms you are having, called *Mold Warriors*." This came just at the right time, which to this day I believe was divine intervention. She went on to explain that the book was about the illness that is caused by indoor toxic mold. I called a mold remediation company the next day and was referred to a professional mold inspector who came out to my house and performed air quality testing in my house. In forty-eight hours I learned that my basement had 5,500 spores of aspergillus/penicillium species per cubic meter. 1500 spores per cubic meter of the same mold was found upstairs and the outside registered about 200. This type of mold is one of the toxic molds that contain dangerous mycotoxins on its spores.

So we gutted the entire basement and tore up and rebuilt both upstairs bathrooms. When they ripped out the moldy fiberglass insulation in the basement ceiling, I developed swelling in my throat that made me feel like I could not breathe, sending me to the emergency room for treatment. I knew that I could not stay at home until renovations were completed. Either I stayed in hotels with Sam or on warm nights we slept in a tent on our back screen porch. I noticed the longer I stayed away from the house, the better I felt. My husband found this time very stressful. He worried that I might not ever be able to live in our house again.

But, soon, I started getting symptoms again. But it was only on days that I worked. What in the world was going on? In the next week it became very clear that work definitely brought on symptoms. The two days a week at work were days that I felt much worse. So I began to suspect my workplace was contaminated with mold as well! This seemed unbelievable to me. What are the odds of both my workplace and home being invaded by toxic mold? I could not believe the newly remodeled office could be moldy. We did not see mold, but I often noticed a slightly moldy smell. I got permission from the owners of my practice to do an air quality test, despite what everyone else thought of the idea. I had it done on my day off. I wore a face mask to protect myself because the previous day at work I could barely breathe and my lungs had been aching by the end of the day. That really scared me.

So, with everyone in the office watching the loopy doctor who had finally gone round the bend, I walked in, mask on, with the mold inspector and had the air in my patient exam room tested. I had to wait two days for the results. The following day, I worked with a mask on, explaining to curious patients that I was allergic to something in the office. I worked until noon, and then took off my mask to eat lunch. That turned out to be a mistake because that half-hour of exposure was enough to throw me into symptoms again. I quickly began to feel short of breath, anxious, weak in the legs and had that strange feeling that I was going to pass out. I told my nurse, that I could not work in the building and would see my next two patients outside. But after the second patient, the owners of my practice caught wind of what was going on and told me just to leave for the day because they could not have me showing patients that there was something wrong with the air in the building, setting them up for a lawsuit. I thought to myself, "But there is something wrong with the air in the building and perhaps tomorrow we will find out what it is!"

At this point, I was beginning to doubt if anything would be found and I was starting to think that maybe I was crazy after all. I went home depressed and felt like I was close to losing my job.

The next day I was tense all morning. Everything stemmed on the results of that test including my sanity, my theory that mold was causing my symptoms and my idea to write a book about this whole ordeal if it did turn out to be mold. My whole world seemed to be wrapped up in this one test.

At a little after 12:00 noon, I got the call from the mold inspector. He said that he had the results of the test back. He had this way of talking that sounded like he was reporting bad news. But I was shocked to hear his next sentence. He said very flatly that the results showed high levels of stachybotrys in the air and the levels shot up to 9000 spores per cubic meter with the HVAC system on. I was speechless. I was expecting toxic mold but I was expecting to find aspergillus or some other less toxic mold but not the dreaded stachybotrys, the most toxic of all the toxic molds. And the levels were very high. I thanked the inspector and as soon as I hung up the phone, I picked up Sam, my seventeen-month-old baby, and started shouting, "We found it, Sam! That's why I have been so sick for so long. No wonder I had been sick. I am lucky to be alive with 9000 spores per cubic meter blowing in my face every five minutes!" One source reports that only a small amount (1mg) of stachybotrys toxin could kill a large horse! And just recently the TV show *Extreme Home Makeover* had featured a family of five who had lost their firefighter father to the black mold, stachybotrys, that he was exposed to while renovating their basement.

Little Sam squealed with delight at seeing me so happy and cheering. It had to have been hard for him, seeing his mom so sick all the time. He could not talk yet, but toddlers can pick up on a lot of things going on around them.

I think I danced around the house for a few hours with Sam that day, celebrating the fact that I was not crazy. I kind of felt like Jimmy Stewart in the movie *It's a Wonderful Life* in the scene where he runs around town after he gets his life back. I called everyone I knew who had known about my mysterious symptoms and told them the "good" news.

The following day, although I was still grateful to have found the answer to my mysterious health problems, reality hit me. First of all, I still had mold toxicity and a large set of symptoms to deal with. I had also developed a nasty sinus infection with bronchitis. I still had tremors, a flu-like feeling, burning pains in my legs, headaches and weakness. These were all symptoms of mold toxicity as described in the book I was reading called *Mold Warriors*. Another curious symptom described in his book is that the symptoms of mold toxicity change from day to day or week to week but there is never a day without symptoms. For the mold toxic individual, that is the most maddening thing about this syndrome, and it makes it appear to other people that you are just plain nuts.

Dr. Ritchie Shoemaker's clinical research and book, *Mold Warriors*, helped give me my life back. His work has uncovered the truth behind mold illness. It's the biotoxins on the mold spores that get into the body and cause the many symptoms of this devastating syndrome. According to his observations and clinical research, about 25% of the population has a particular HLA genotype that somehow makes it impossible for the body to recognize and excrete these biotoxins. So they accumulate and the longer you are exposed, the sicker you get. He has treated over 2000 toxic mold syndrome patients from all over the country. There is a medication he has tremendous success with called cholestyramine. It is an old cholesterol medication that has been used for many years with few side effects. It binds to the biotoxins as they pass through the intestinal tract. Once the toxins bind to the cholestyramine you've got them. They don't get reabsorbed back into the bloodstream but pass out harmlessly through the intestines. Without cholestyramine, the biotoxins, which go anywhere just looking for some nerves to attack, will circulate through the intestines and just get reabsorbed back into the bloodstream. It takes about two to four weeks of cholestyramine at one packet four times daily on an empty stomach. Dr Shoemaker claims to have a high success rate of about 90% of people that take cholestyramine, returning to a normal and symptom free life. He notices also that all of his toxic mold patients are primed for mold sensitivity for the rest of their lives. For example, a person who has had mold illness, even though completely recovered, could walk into a moldy building and immediately, or in a few hours, experience symptoms again. These symptoms again abate once cholestyramine is administered. The good news is that once armed with this knowledge, former toxic mold sufferers won't let themselves fall into the "mold trap" again. They will know by their symptoms that they are being exposed to toxic mold and they will be able to take the proper action necessary to protect themselves. Whether it be changing jobs, changing hotels on vacation, or frequenting only restaurants, stores and gyms that don't bring on symptoms.

Buildings both commercial and residential can have toxic mold. And it isn't only old buildings. In fact some of the newer construction can be the worst! Many people in the market to buy houses only look at newer construction to avoid mold and don't realize that newer buildings might be more likely to have mold problems due to sloppy construction practices. In an effort to get the job done fast, corners may be cut. New construction may use green wood that has moisture in it. Siding may be slapped up over wood that had been rained on and not allowed to dry. Insulation left out in the rain, may be put into walls before being allowed to dry. Leaky roofs and bad plumbing can cause water intrusion. All these mistakes spell out mold disasters for the new homeowners. And these unlucky people won't even know what is making them sick. They will spend thousands of dollars seeing doctors trying to figure out what is wrong, while it is the house itself that is slowly sickening them.

In the weeks that followed my positive mold test, I stopped working. I would not risk continued exposure to toxic mold. I needed to recover. Upon leaving the office my symptoms were shortness of breath, aching lungs, weakness in my legs, anxiety, flu-like symptoms, and fatigue. Gradually the shortness of breath resolved along with the lungs aching. The symptoms changed to tremors, difficulty walking, anxiety and burning muscle pains in my thighs. The tremors gradually resolved and then I had very severe fatigue. It was a struggle just to move, not to mention chasing after my very active, now eighteen-month-old toddler. Along with the fatigue the muscle aches got worse. When these two symptoms resolved, the panic attacks returned. The feeling that I was going to pass out was the hallmark of my panic attacks, along with a racing heart rate and weakness. With all these other symptoms, headaches would come and go. Sharp stabbing fleeting ice-pick like pains would appear anywhere in my body, at any time. The muscle pains concentrated in my thighs as a burning aching pain.

I was feeling awful. The best way I can describe chronic neurotoxicity from toxic mold is that you feel that you are dying very slowly and painfully. It is hard to describe if you have never felt it before. I have never experienced anything like it before in my life. In my opinion, no one can know just what it is like unless they experience it themselves.

After about two weeks of being away from my workplace and taking quite a bit of cholestyramine, my symptoms had lessened. Then I started to develop sores in my mouth, which is a side effect of the medication, so I had to stop for a while. A few weeks later I continued on the cholestyramine program. Immediately after starting just one dose, I noticed some improvement. Then gradually over a period of four months, my symptoms subsided.

The neurological symptoms and the sensation that I was going to pass out were too terrifying to consider returning to work. The prospect of losing my health if I kept my job was simply not worth the money. I decided my health was more important for myself, and my family. It is a shame that in today's world, I would be forced to make that choice.

With the safety of my work environment still in question, I knew I had to look for work somewhere else. I explored applying for workman's compensation but in order to do that I had to pay $6000 out of pocket to cover testing that my insurance would not cover. They would not give me a referral out of network to the only doctor in Michigan that treats mold illness. Instead my insurance plan wanted to throw me to the wolves by sending me to their doctor in network who deals with mold illness, who also happened to be the doctor who regularly testifies against mold victims for the insurance companies. Would that have been fair?

So not having the money to sue for workman's compensation, coupled with the huge expenses we just had remediating our house and then added to my loss of income from not being able to work, we suffered much financial loss. My husband, being a schoolteacher, counted on my income to afford our house. We thought we might be able to keep our house, using money in savings. When you save your money for a rainy day, this is what they are talking about. This was a rainy day.

There are no laws to protect citizens from toxic indoor mold. I called the Environmental Protection Agency (EPA) and found out they cannot protect us because there are no laws in place. I called OSHA and found out they do not have anything to do with mold in the workplace. At the top of their claim form they state they do not handle mold problems. I called the health department and they could not do anything to help me, either. Building owners can do what they please because there are no laws to protect the public from toxic mold.

In retrospect, I can say that the vast majority of my symptoms were due to stachybotrys and chaetomium exposure at my workplace. Before moving to the new office I had some typical allergy symptoms along with sinus inflammation and dizziness. I was being exposed both at home and at the old workplace to aspergillus and penicillium molds. But it was not until moving into our new office building that I began to experience the neurological symptoms that felt like multiple sclerosis like the shaking, trouble walking and difficulty focusing my eyes as well as the panic attacks and generalized anxiety.

Today, I am about 90% recovered. I still experience some anxiety spells and setbacks from time to time and hope that, someday, that will be completely diminished to a level I enjoyed before the mold exposure. I am still working on detoxifying using the different treatments I have listed in this book. It is a gradual process that I am confident will result in improved health. I am careful to keep toxic mold out of my life. My nose usually lets me know when I am in a building that has mold in it and I get out if I can. I keep a dehumidifier running at all times in my basement and I use a HEPA filter in my house in the cold weather. In the summer, all the windows are kept open and fans are always on. I continue on the Healing diet as much as possible, and take a lot of antioxidants, probiotics and a brown seaweed detoxification supplement called Limu Moui as well as the general supplements I recommend. If I stray too much from the Healing diet and the supplements, some symptoms return, but resolve as soon as I resume the program. I work as a family practice physician, specializing in nutrition and the detoxification of toxic black mold syndrome.

Chapter 2
What Is Toxic Mold?

Before my experience with toxic black mold, I did not know that indoor molds could be toxic. I was familiar with the mycotoxin called aflatoxin, that is found in foods like peanuts and carrots. But I was not aware that toxic indoor molds could spew out thousands of toxic spores that would make people sick upon inhalation.

Toxic mold is simply mold that produces large amounts of toxins on the spores that it releases into the air. All molds produce spores as a way of reproducing. The spores are like the seeds or the offspring of the mold. So to protect their precious children, the mold covers the spores in toxins to prevent the spore from being eaten and to compete with other molds and bacteria. Spores are very hardy also. They can usually withstand extremes of temperature, chemicals and even boiling sometimes. Enough toxin-laden spores can kill large animals. One mg of stachybotrys toxin can kill a large horse. Spores are very small, in fact, microscopic. It is estimated that 6000 spores can fit on the head of a pin. The toxins are extremely potent so that even at these small doses, toxic molds are extremely dangerous. It is believed that some of these toxins might have been used in biological warfare.

How Do Toxic Molds Make Us Sick?

They make us sick by poisoning us with the mycotoxins that are on their spores and fungal fragments. These mycotoxins are potent biotoxins. These mycotoxins can accumulate in the body so that, the longer the exposure, the more toxic a person becomes. Mycotoxins cause inflammation in the body and that is how they create symptoms. Apparently, some people are better than others at excreting these toxins. According to the clinical research of Dr. Shoemaker and another study, 25% of the population have a certain genotype that makes them more susceptible to mold toxicity. It is theorized that this is because they cannot excrete biotoxins very efficiently. But even a person who is not mold susceptible can get sick from exposure to a high concentration of mycotoxins. Generally the people that get better gradually after leaving a moldy building, without any help from medication, are the non-mold susceptible people (about 75% of the population). And the people that do not get better upon leaving a moldy building, and only get better with help from medication are the unlucky mold susceptible (25% of the population). One of the most frustrating things about this illness is that not everyone in a moldy building gets that sick! The 75% (non-mold susceptible people) do get sick, but not as bad, because whenever they leave the building, their bodies start detoxifying. The 25% (mold susceptible people) do not detoxify upon leaving the building, so the toxins just keep on building up in their bodies until they get very sick. The 25% that do get sick are looked upon as oddities because they are in the minority. In this era of minority rights and such, this can be looked upon as a form of discrimination against minorities. Are the 25% to suffer because 75% don't understand? Lawyers testifying against mold victims frequently use this phenomenon to try to discredit the mold susceptible person. They point out that not everyone in the moldy building got sick; therefore, it had to be something else that caused their illness.

Indoor Mold Versus Outdoor Mold

Toxic mold is generally indoor mold. Some toxic mold can exist outdoors, but because of the vast competition in nature, they cannot grow into large colonies. Outdoors, molds use most of their energy just to survive rather than to reproduce. So they do not put out a large number of spores. The only condition in which molds spew out a huge amount of spores is in a warm moist environment with no competition. This is called amplified growth and it only occurs indoors.

So when lawyers in toxic mold cases use the argument that molds are everywhere so why would they be a problem now, indoors, the rebuttal should be that indoor molds have amplified growth. And with amplified growth conditions, toxic molds grow more than non-toxic molds. Amplified growth also encourages molds to spew out much more toxin-laden spores.

The types of toxic molds and the mycotoxins they produce are as follows:

Penicillium species

Mycotoxins produced include:

Ochratoxin A, which causes cancer and kidney disease.
Patulin, which causes cancer, swelling, internal bleeding and paralysis and convulsions.
Penicillic acid, which causes liver damage, kidney damage, cancer and swelling.
Penitrem, which causes tremors, muscle dysfunction and death.
Other mycotoxins produced by penicillium are anacine, arisugacins A&B, Auranthine (sclerotigenin), aurantiamine, belfedrin A, botryodiplodin, brevianamid A, chaetoglobosin A, B & C, Chlororugulovasines A&B, chrysogine, citromycetin, etc. The list goes on and is very extensive.

Aspergillus Species

There are several types of aspergillus, namely:

Aspergillus ochraceous
Aspergillus clavatus
Aspergillus niger
Aspergillus versicolor

This mold type can be found in building insulation, fireproofing material, soil, grains, dead leaves, and grass. A study in 1994 found that fiberglass insulation is susceptible to fungal colonization especially by Aspergillus versicolor, only when relative humidity exceeded 50%.

The mycotoxins produced by this group include:

Aflatoxin:
This is the most carcinogenic substance known to man, and it is produced by the ochraceous type of aspergillus. In cattle it suppresses appetite, causes weight loss and decreases milk production. In humans it can cause jaundice, liver damage, abdominal pain, gastrointestinal bleeding and death.

Cyclopiazonic acid:
This mycotoxin can cause anorexia, diarrhea, dehydration, weight loss, paralysis, hemorrhaging and death.

Tremorgens::
In humans this mycotoxin can cause fatigue, headaches, fever, chills, nausea, vomiting, tremors and dementia.

Tricothecenes:
These mycotoxins suppress the immune system and can cause abdominal pain, vomiting, diarrhea, bloody stools and facial rash.

Stachybotrys Species

Mycotoxins produced include satratoxin H, trichoverrol, and cyclosporins. These mycotoxins suppress the immune system, affecting the lymphoid tissue and bone marrow and can cause kidney and liver cancer. Symptoms of exposure include dermatitis, cough, nosebleed, rhinitis, headaches, fatigue, flu-like symptoms, burning in the mouth and nose, and fever.

Trichothecenes are the most well known class of toxins produced by stachybotrys. They are produced by other molds too. They are potent protein inhibitors and are thought to be the cause of the pulmonary hemorrhaging seen in poisoning from stachybotrys.

Stachybotrys is a greenish-black slimy mold that grows under conditions of high moisture. It does not grow on concrete, linoleum or tiles. It is not the mold that grows on bathroom shower tiles. It has to have some kind of cellulose product to live on such as wood or paper.

Scopulariopsis Species

The mycotoxins for this mold are unknown.

Fusarium Species

This mold can be found in corn and corn products. Its mycotoxin, fumonisin, has been linked to birth defects because it may interfere with utilization of folic acid.

Also tricothecenes mycotoxins are produced by this mold.

Chaetomium

This mold can cause onychomycosis (nail fungus infections) and is highly opportunistic in cancer patients. It is thought that this mold can cause neurological damage that may be irreversible.

Produces the mycotoxins, sterigmatocystin and chaetomium.

As you can see, the amount of different types of mycotoxins on spores is enormous. And most of the toxins have not been studied and the effects on the human body are unknown. Some of the mycotoxins can cause cancer while others may cause temporary or permanent neurological damage and birth defects like spina bifida. Some mycotoxins have been used to help humans such as antibiotics (i.e. penicillin) and ergot alkaloids for headaches and hemorrhaging.

Chapter 3
The Mold Allergy Versus Mold Toxin Controversy

There is a controversy over whether exposure to toxic mold causes a plain old allergic reaction or symptoms due to mold toxins accumulating in the body. In plain terms, is it mold allergy or mold toxicity? I believe that based on studies, the unusual symptoms of toxic black mold syndrome are the result of a buildup of mycotoxins in the body. Yes, I do also believe that like any other mold, there can be allergic reactions as well. But the unusual symptoms are due to toxicity of the mold toxins and not to allergies.

First of all, let's examine why this controversy has arisen in the first place. I think it has come about because not everyone, due to genetic differences among individuals, experiences the toxic effects of mold exposure. However, there is a percentage of the population who do experience the toxic effect of toxic mold. This was shown clearly in a study appearing in the *Annals of Allergy, Asthma and Immunology* by Edmondson and Fink at the Medical College of Wisconsin. They found that out of 36 children and 29 adults who believed they had toxic mold syndrome, most were only experiencing allergy symptoms. But, 25% of that group had what the author described as "symptoms not compatible with allergy." The patients in this study had symptoms ranging from runny nose and cough to shortness of breath, wheezing, chest tightness, itchy eyes, nosebleed, urinary problems, nausea, vomiting, abdominal pain and nervous system problems such as dizziness, anxiety, weakness, restless legs, memory loss, and shaking.

Certainly symptoms of memory loss, anxiety, shaking, nausea and vomiting that the 25% of the subjects in this study were experiencing are not typical allergy symptoms. There has to be another explanation for people exposed to toxic black mold experiencing these non-allergic symptoms.

An article published on the front page of the January 9, 2007 issue of *The Wall Street Journal*, titled "Amid Suits Over Mold, Experts Wear Two Hats" addresses the issue of this controversy over toxic mold syndrome. Apparently, lawyers involved in defending against toxic mold litigation cases frequently refer to a position paper from The American College of Occupational and Environmental Medicine (ACOEM) which states that "scientific evidence does not support the proposition that human health has been adversely affected by inhaled mycotoxins in the home, school or office environment."

This statement, from ACOEM's position paper, has been used very successfully by lawyers working for builders, landlords and insurers as an important defense strategy in toxic mold cases. David Armstrong, the investigator in this story and author of this *Wall Street Journal* article, goes on to state that this position paper was written by people who are regular paid experts for mold litigation defendants. Talk about a conflict of interest! It's no wonder it is so difficult these days to win a toxic mold case.

According to this article, ACOEM does not disclose in its paper that the authors are paid experts in mold litigation, and the president of the organization claims no disclosure is needed because the paper is a statement from their society as a whole and not just the authors of the article. So, ACOEM as a whole supports this statement despite the study cited previously showing 25% of the subjects have symptoms that cannot be explained by typical allergies. Two authors of the ACOEM statement were paid 375 to 500 dollars an hour to testify on the defense side in mold cases. A third author gets paid 500 to 720 dollars per hour on the defense side in mold cases.

ACOEM knew about the authors' conflicts of interest and internal documents circulating at ACOEM showed that they were concerned about the paper being too slanted towards defendants in toxic mold cases.

Also The American Academy of Allergy, Asthma and Immunology published a position paper that states that it is highly unlikely that enough mycotoxins could be inhaled to lead to toxic health effects. However it was found that, in this case also, two of its authors were paid defense experts in mold litigation. The academy later included a disclosure in their position paper that two authors were paid experts on the defense side of mold litigation cases.

All of this, is part of the reason why the medical community is not recognizing toxic mold syndrome. When a prestigious organization such as ACOEM comes out and basically says toxic mold syndrome does not exist, people take it as gospel truth. But when people see the conflict of interest that is involved, they may reconsider whether to believe the position that this organization is taking on this subject. If you look at the evidence, it's obvious that there is a toxic component to toxic black mold syndrome. Yes there is an allergic component to the syndrome…of course, it's a mold and people can be allergic to it, just like any other mold and develop normal allergic reactions to it. But it is a TOXIN as well, and in some people it does accumulate and cause toxic effects.

In my case, I have had allergies all my life and have never experienced the symptoms I had upon exposure to stachybotrys and chaetomium. How can someone say that shaking, anxiety, panic attacks, burning pains in my thighs, weakness, memory loss and near syncopal episodes are allergic symptoms? Even a non-physician knows that these symptoms are not due to allergies.

The evidence for mold toxicity is here. Research does support the toxicity of toxic molds.

One recent study in 2006 found that satratoxin G, the toxin found in stachybotrys caused loss of sensory neurons in the nose and inflammation in the brains and noses of mice, suggesting that this toxin is neurotoxic and can cause inflammation in the nasal passages and brains of those exposed to these toxins.

In another study, rats fed corn infested with fifty-three different species of chaetomium, twenty-five of those species killed the rats within four to five days.

In 1983, ducks fed T-2 mycotoxins had a drop in weight, developed caseonecrotic plaques in their ailimentary tracts and severe ulcerative proliferative esphagitis and proventiculitis. Also they developed atrophy of all their lymphoid tissue.

A study in 1983 showed lambs fed T-2 mycotoxins developed decreased white blood cell count and lymphocyte count and atrophy of the lymph tissue.

In 1983, a study found that one hundred sheep that died on a Hungarian farm had been exposed to satratoxin G from stachybotrys atra contamination of their straw bedding.

One study in 2000 found that a single potent exposure to stachybotrys chartarum spores resulted in inflammation and injury to the lungs of rats. This study also showed that this effect was dose dependent and definitely due to the toxins present on the spores.

Other studies have demonstrated the toxicity of mycotoxins.

In one study, trichothecene mycotoxins, satratoxin H and G and trichoverrols A and B were found to be on the spores of stachybotyrs atra and were found to strongly inhibit protein synthesis. Also, in the same study it was found that particles of fungus including spores were less than 15 microns in diameter, thus making them able to be breathed right into the lungs. This study demonstrates that inhalation of aerosolized spores of stachybotrys could be quite dangerous.

A 1999 article in Environmental Health Perspectives states that diseases associated with inhalation of fungal spores includes toxic pneumonitis, hypersensitivity pneumonitis, tremors, chronic fatigue syndrome, kidney failure, and cancer.

Another study in 2002 identified stachylysin as the possible toxin produced by stachybotrys that caused the cases of pulmonary hemosiderosis in infants in Cleveland, Ohio.

One case of a young man who developed a neurological syndrome called, tremorgenic encephalopathy including tremors and dementia following exposure to a moldy silo on a farm. Symptoms resolved completely in one week. It is speculated that his illness was due to exposure to a tremorgenic mycotoxin.

Another case described a farmer and his wife who developed temporary respiratory distress after being in moldy granary for eight hours. The next day the wife developed acute renal failure, which eventually resolved in twenty-four days. A strain of Aspergillus ochraceus producing the mycotoxin, ochratoxin was isolated from the wheat in the granary. In this same article the speculation that the mysterious deaths of archaeologists that had opened the Egyptian tombs was due to inhalation of mycotoxins was discussed. This hypothesis has not been verified.

A study in 1996 showed that amongst office workers in a water-damaged building, there were reports of respiratory, central nervous system, mucous membrane disorders and a possible immune competency dysfunction demonstrated by abnormalities in cellular and humoral immune system parameters.

In a study in 1987, inhalation of T-2 mycotoxins in mice was at least ten times more toxic than systemic administration of the mycotoxin. Inhalation was found to be twenty times more toxic than skin absorption of mycotoxins.

A study in 2004 showed a significant number of occupants of mold-contaminated buildings tested positive for stachybotrys exposure through an ELISA test that was highly specific for macrocyclic trichothecenes. This study demonstrated that tricothecene mycotoxins can be found in some people exposed to stachybotrys through ELISA testing of the blood. I do not know of a lab that uses this method of testing.

Acute pulmonary hemorrhage in infants in Cleveland, Ohio, in 1991 has been shown by epidemiologic evidence to be associated with exposure to stachybotrys in water-damaged housing. According to an article in *Current Opinions in Pediatrics,* by Ruth A. Etzel, the amount of research in the area of stachybotrys causing pulmonary hemorrhaging shows strength, consistency, coherence and specificity. Advances in the understanding of this have occurred through animal models, biologic mechanism of injury, dose-response relationships, isolation of mold from diseased patients, detection methods and intervention.

The mycotoxins of toxic molds belong to a class of naturally occurring toxins called biotoxins. Other biotoxins include the venom of brown recluse and yellowsac (household) spiders, ciguatera and pfiesteria fish poisoning, toxic blue green algaes and Lyme spirochetes. The symptoms from poisoning, from these sources is documented. The symptoms of poisoning from ciguatera are very similar to the symptoms described by toxic black mold victims. Primarily the ciguatera biotoxins affect the nervous system and gastrointestinal tract. Sound familiar? Nervous symptoms include parasthesias numbness tingling burning and pain, temperature reversal, vertigo, dental pain, blurred vision, tremors, psychiatric problems and pain on urination. Gastrointestinal complaints include nausea, vomiting, diarrhea, abdominal pain and cramping. Also there can be fatigue weakness arthralgias, breathing problems, myalgias, heart arrhythmias, racing heart rate, low blood pressure, headache and metallic taste in the mouth. There can be cases of symptoms for only a few days or one to even several years. Since this sounds so familiar to toxic black mold syndrome, and toxic molds produce mycotoxins that belong to a general class of natural toxins called biotoxins, does it not follow that toxic mold syndrome could be a result of accumulation in the body of these biotoxins produced by mold? It seems so simple yet why there is even a controversy does not actually make any scientific sense. The arguments some people make is that the amount of mycotoxin-laden spores that someone would breath in is so low that it could not possibly cause symptoms. Well, guess what, it has! And that statement is, by the way, ridiculous to say if you have no idea how many spores someone is breathing in. In my case, I was getting about 9000 spores per cubic meter. I would like to challenge the group who made the statement that someone could not be exposed to enough toxins to make a difference. Maybe they would like to try being exposed to 9000 spores of stachybotrys per cubic meter every five minutes and see how they feel a week later. That would make believers out of them really fast.

Chapter 4
Mycotoxins in History

There are about four hundred different mycotoxins that are produced by molds. Throughout history there have been many cases of mycotoxins causing both human and animal illnesses and death. Mycotoxins can cause harm through ingestion in contaminated foods, inhalation of toxic spores and dermal exposure to toxic spores.

Ergot alkaloids are mycotoxins produced by the mold claviceps purpura and played a prominent role in mycotoxin-induced illness in the Middle Ages. This type of mycotoxin contamination affected rye grains in those days. Two different types of ergot poisoning existed; gangrenous and convulsive. In the gangrenous form, an initial prickly sensation in a limb was followed by swelling, searing pain, and sensations of intense hot and cold. That's why this syndrome was called St Anthony's Fire. Continued vasoconstriction by the ergot led to loss of limbs due to gangrene. Convulsive ergotism is characterized by convulsions, hallucinations and other nervous system symptoms. Today, ergot poisoning is rare. Ergot alkaloids are used medically, today, to treat migraine headaches and control post-partum hemorrhage.

Timeline for Mycotoxins in History

In the Old Testament of the Bible, in Leviticus 14:33, God warns the Israelites about mold in houses. In Leviticus 14:34-53, "leprous plague" is translated as decomposition by mildew, mold, dry rot, etc. So, in the following excerpt I have replaced the word "leprous plague" with "mold" or "mold infestation."

And the Lord spoke to Moses and Aaron, saying: When you come into the land of Canaan, which I give you as a possession, and I put the mold infestation in a house in the land of your possession, and he who owns the house comes and tells the priest, saying, It seems to me there is some mold in the house, then the priest shall command that they empty the house, before the priest goes into it to examine the mold, that all that is in the house may not be made unclean; and afterward the priest shall go in to examine the house.

And he shall examine the mold: and indeed if the mold is on the walls of the house with ingrained streaks, greenish or reddish, which appear to be deep in the wall, then the priest shall go out of the house, to the door of the house and shut up the house seven days And the priest shall come again on the seventh day and look and indeed if the mold has spread on the walls of the house, the priest shall command that they take away the stones in which is the mold, and they shall cast them into an unclean place outside the city.

And he shall cause the house to be scraped inside, all around, and the dust that they scrape off they shall pour out in an unclean place outside the city.

Then they shall take other stones and put them into the place of those stones, and he shall take other mortar and plaster the house.

Now if the mold comes back and breaks out in the house, after he has taken away the stones, after he has scraped the house, and after it is plastered, then the priest shall come and look: and indeed if the mold has spread in the house, it is an active mold in the house. It is unclean.

And he shall break down the house, its stones, its timber, and all the plaster of the house, and he shall carry them outside the city to an unclean place.

Moreover, he who goes into the house at all while it is shut up shall be unclean until evening. And he who lies down in the house shall wash his clothes and he who eats in the house shall wash his clothes.

But if the priest comes in and examines it, and indeed the mold has not spread in the house after the house was plastered, then the priest shall pronounce the house clean, because the mold is healed.

430 B.C.

The plague of Athens is theorized to have been caused by ingestion of T-2 mycotoxins.

Sixth Century B.C.
The Assyrians poisoned enemy wells with rye ergot.

Middle Ages: 9th to 14th century
Gangrenous ergot poisoning (St Anthony's Fire) from eating contaminated rye grains.

16th to 19th century Europe
Convulsive ergot poisoning from eating contaminated rye grains.

1692 New England
The Salem Witch Trials are now thought by historians to be caused by ergot poisoning. The convulsions and hallucinations experienced by suspected witches were caused by ingestion of contaminated rye grains.

1942 to 1948
100,000 deaths in the Orenburg district of Russia were caused by eating wheat and corn that had been under the snow for the winter and had become contaminated with fusarium and stachybotyrs molds. During World War II, the men of this village were fighting the war and had left the corn and wheat in the fields over the winter. In the spring the corn and wheat were harvested, but were contaminated with mold. The disease produced by consumption of these moldy grains was called alimentary toxic aleukia and is characterized by necrotic ulcers in the nose, mouth, throat, stomach, and intestines, and sometimes hemorrhage from the nose, mouth, GI tract, and kidneys. The mortality rate was 10-60%. In the 1940s Soviet scientists gave the name stachybotrytoxicosis to the set of symptoms following inhalation of the stachybotyrs mycotoxins, which are sore throat, bloody nose, shortness of breath, cough, low grade fever, and chest tightness.

1961 to 1985 China
Many outbreaks of vomiting following consumption of vomitoxin contaminated grains. Vomitoxin or deoxynvatenol is a tricothecene mycotoxin found in stachybotyrs, fusarium and other molds.

1970s to 1980s
There is controversy whether or not an aerosolized T2 tricothecene mycotoxin called yellow rain was used as biological warfare, killing 6300 in

Laos during the Vietnam War. Also, there are reports of uses of T-2 mycotoxins in Kampuchea and Afghanistan in 1979 to 1981.

1987 India
100 people became ill after eating wheat products containing the mycotoxin, vomitoxin.

1989-1990
There were many cases of Fatal equine (horse) leukomalacia and porcine (pig) pulmonary edema in U.S., caused by fumonisin contaminated corn products.

1990
A cluster of neural tube defects in South Texas is postulated to be caused by high ingestion of fumonisin contaminated corn products amongst Mexican Americans. Fumonisin is a mycotoxin that interferes with cellular uptake of folic acid and this might be why folic acid supplementation in this group did not protect those women from birth defects.

1997 to 1998
1700 U.S. children became sick with vomiting, nausea, headaches and abdominal cramps following ingestion of burritos containing low levels of vomitoxins. The levels were low for adults but might have been too much for children.

1994
Pulmonary hemorrhaging in infants in housing contaminated with stachybotyrs in Cleveland, Oho.

1998
A courthouse and two associated buildings were contaminated with stachybotrys chartarum and aspergillus versicolor and caused illness in its inhabitants. Those with symptoms had new onset psychiatric symptoms that began only after the mold exposure.

2002
Stachybotrys and other mold contamination of a conference center in Columbia, Maryland. 45 of 55 conference employees became ill.

There have been many present-day cases of toxic mold syndrome including the deceased firefighter featured on *Extreme Home Makeover*, Erin Brockovich, Bianca Jagger, and Ed McMahon.

There are most likely many cases in New Orleans, following the extensive flooding from hurricane Katrina.

In the present day, with the increase in global warming that is causing a dramatic change in weather patterns, there could be more mold growth and mold related illnesses. Drought and flooding both can cause problems with increased mold and mycotoxins. Drought can weaken the plant so that fungus can penetrate seed kernels. Flooding causes increased water in the environment, which can cause mold growth and resultant mycotoxin contamination. We see an example of this today in New Orleans, as thousands of homes are water damaged and thus mold contaminated. And with the humidity levels in New Orleans, it will be hard to control any mold that has started growing in a building.

Also, as our buildings get older and repairs may not be made to keep water out, we might be seeing more mold contamination in older poorly repaired buildings. We are seeing this in our nation's school system because of lack of funding in education. Cheaper flat roofs on schools are more prone to leaking. In many cases necessary repairs on school roofs are not being done due to lack of funds. Since mold illness can cause symptoms of attention deficit hyperactivity disorder (ADHD) as well as other symptoms, this problem needs a solution as soon as possible; for the lives of our children.

Chapter 5
Symptoms of Toxic
Black Mold Syndrome

It may seem to some that it's ridiculous how many symptoms can be attributed to toxic black mold syndrome. The reason there are so many different symptoms lies in four important facts. First of all, there are many types of toxic molds and each of these molds produce many different types of mycotoxins. Secondly, each toxic mold generates many and different mycotoxins depending on the environmental conditions. Thirdly, each individual responds differently to these mycotoxins depending on their own specific genetic makeup. Finally, mycotoxins affect the cytokine system of the body, which causes general pain and inflammation in many systems of the body, which can explain the many different symptoms.

So, with all these variables, it's no wonder that this syndrome can present so many different ways. But, because it presents so many different ways, many people jump to the false conclusion that the mold toxic individual is not really sick and is looking for something to blame all his/her problems on. Many have attacked toxic mold syndrome sufferers because they find it so hard to believe that so many symptoms can be attributed to one syndrome.

I was one of those people who had seen reports of people becoming ill from toxic black mold and I hate to admit it now but I really did not believe their stories. I thought they sounded too incredulous to be true especially when they claimed that their symptoms continued well after leaving the mold-infested building. Now I am the victim and I know what it is like to have people doubting the credibility of their story.

The most distinguishing characteristic of this syndrome is that the symptoms change. That is they change from day to day from week to week or month to month. The best explanation for why this occurs seems to be that the toxins migrate through the body attacking different organ systems as they go. This characteristic not only drives the mold toxic individual nearly crazy, but it makes it appear to those observing the whole situation, that he is just, plain nuts. One of my good friends at work, with whom I confided with about my mysterious symptoms, left an article on my desk on hypochondriacs. I know she meant well, but it made me want to scream in frustration.

Another important thing to consider, regarding symptoms, is that if your symptoms cannot be explained by any medical condition, you should consider mold toxicity. In other words, if you have been to doctors and they do not know what is wrong with you, and tests have all come back negative, you need to consider mold toxicity as the cause of your symptoms. If you get a diagnosis of depression and get handed a prescription for an antidepressant as I did, it is possible that what you have is mold toxicity. Many doctors, when they are unsure what is wrong with you, fall back on depression as their waste-basket diagnosis, even when it is well known that the some of the symptoms the patient is complaining of have nothing to do with depression. In my case, the neurological symptoms I was experiencing, I knew had nothing to do with depression. That is not even a controversy in medicine. It is true, however, that depression can cause things like anxiety, panic attacks, and pains. But, still, a lot of the depression, anxiety and pain in our population could at least be partially caused by mold toxins.

So, in summary, there are three important things to remember about the symptoms of mold toxicity.

The symptoms are many and varied depending on the type of mold, the mycotoxin cocktail produced by that type of mold or molds, and your individual response to those mycotoxins.

The symptoms change frequently, sometimes from day to day, week to week or month to month, but never really go away.

The symptoms cannot be explained by a known medical condition. Doctors do not know what is wrong with you, all your tests come back negative and you might have been handed a prescription for an antidepressant.

So with all this having been said, here is a list of possible symptoms that mold exposure can cause. The list starts with the most common symptoms. This list is compiled from many different sources on toxic mold syndrome. Even as extensive as this is, it is always possible that someone may have one not listed here as a result of toxic mold exposure.

Most common symptoms:

- -muscle pain, cramps, burning, unusual shooting (ice pick-like) pains
- -headaches
- -fatigue, weakness, flu-like symptoms, fever, chills
- -shortness of breath, cough
- -abdominal pain, diarrhea
- -chronic sinusitis, sore throat
- -burning eyes, red eyes, sensitivity to light
- -difficulty with thought processes, memory loss, loss of concentration, confusion, disorientation, "brain fog"
- -dizziness
- -metallic taste in mouth
- -numbness and tingling
- -night sweats
- -temperature regulation problems
- -excessive thirst and urination
- -rash
- -excessive menstrual bleeding
- -balance problems
- -mylar flush (face flushing) *I had this, people thought I looked healthy because of it
- -chest pains
- -IgA nephropathy (kidney disease)
- -Increased infections

Other symptoms:

- -the sensation that you are going to pass out
- -panic attacks
- -tremors
- -attention deficit disorder
- -vision problems
- -swollen lymph nodes
- -anxiety, depression
- -difficulty losing weight
- -ringing in the ears
- -hearing loss
- -chronic fatigue

-multiple chemical sensitivity (stachybotrys and chaetomium)
-nose bleeds and pulmonary hemorrhaging (stachybotrys)
-bruising, hives
-infertility, miscarriage
-fibromyalgia
-chronic fatigue
-multiple sclerosis like symptoms
-dirt like taste in mouth
-cancer
-hair loss
-joint pains
-irregular heart beat
-heart attack
-seizure
-muscle twitching
-anaphylaxis on re-exposure to toxic molds
-air hunger, can't get a deep breath
-child development delays
-lateness
-apathy
-difficulty handling any kind of stress
-mood swings, irritability
-frequent upper respiratory infections
-sensitivity to sound
-nausea, vomiting
-new food allergies
-jaundice (yellowing of the skin or eyes)
-poor insight into illness
-stomach ulcers
-death, in extreme cases (Firefighter father of five featured on 2006 episode of *Extreme Home Makeover*)

As you can see these toxins affect the brain. That is because most are neurotoxins. One interesting effect these neurotoxins seem to have on the frontal lobe of the brain, according to one source, is a poor insight into one's illness and thus an unwillingness to do anything about one's plight. It's almost like the mold toxins are paralyzing the brain into apathy. Sounds like a creepy science fiction movie, doesn't it? I have observed this symptom myself in some mold-affected people.

Chapter 6
Diagnosis of Toxic
Black Mold Syndrome

First of all, in order to be diagnosed with toxic black mold syndrome, I am sorry to say that you are probably going to have to diagnose yourself. Many doctors will find fault with this statement especially since I myself am a physician. However, desperate times call for desperate measures and the truth is most doctors do not know how to recognize or treat toxic black mold syndrome. In fact, the medical profession still does not think it really exists. Many are still of the belief that it is just normal allergy even though evidence shows in studies that 25% of those exposed to toxic mold have symptoms not attributed to normal allergies. You might be able to find an environmental physician that can recognize this condition, but they might just treat it as an allergy, which does not work to remove mold toxins. But it helps to get the diagnosis and then you can treat it yourself with the help of your family physician.

So, the options are:

1. Find an environmental physician in your area. To locate one call: ACOEM (American College of Occupational and Environmental Medicine)

www.acoem.org
25 Northwest Point Blvd.
Suite 700
Elk Grove Village, Illinois 60007-1030
(847) 818-1800

or

National Association of Mold Professionals (NAMP)
3250 Old Farm Lane, Suite 1
Walled Lake, MI 48390
(248) 669-5673
www.moldpro.org

2. Diagnose Yourself

A. Determine if your symptoms match up with the criteria in the previous symptom chapter. *Yes*

B. Determine if the onset of your symptoms correlates with a known mold exposure or a new building exposure or new house. *Yes*

C. Obtain IAQ (indoor air quality) testing of places you live and work to find out what you are breathing in your air. There are several ways of testing your environment for mold and these are explained in the chapter on testing. *did*

D. Determine if leaving the suspected moldy building leads to an improvement in symptoms. This test can be unreliable because 75% of the population will have an improvement in symptoms on leaving a moldy building, but 25% of the population will not have a significant improvement in symptoms because they do not detoxify from the mold toxins as quickly. I have seen some people use this as a test, and decide prematurely that mold must not be their problem since leaving the moldy building does not help. So this test should be used with the knowledge that it is not at all reliable.

E. Visual Contrast Sensitivity is a vision test that tests for biotoxins in the body. Its patented name is Functional Acuity Contrast Test FACT (Stereo Optical Co., Inc. Chicago IL US Patent #s 4,365,873 & 5,414,479). This test measures visual contrast sensitivity which is decreases upon exposure to mold toxins. The diagnostic chart is available for doctors to order at a cost of $275.

You can also take the test yourself online for a small fee of 8.95 per test. The website is www.chronicneurotoxins.com and is the website provided by Dr. Ritchie Shoemaker, M.D., author of *Mold Warriors*. It is an easy test to take that just involves looking at lines and determining the direction of the lines.

F. There is a laboratory that specializes in mold testing using DNA probes of tissue or body fluids. They have DNA probes for the many different types of toxic molds. These tests do not test the blood, but test the urine, nasal washes or nasal secretions for the presence of toxic molds. This lab also performs testing for three of the most common mycotoxins, which are ochratoxin, aflatoxin and tricothecenes. For these tests they need either samples of first morning urine, nasal washes or nasal secretions. The presence of these mycotoxins in the urine and nasal secretions, has been found to correlate with toxic mold exposure. These tests are the best way I know of testing for exposure to toxic molds.

This lab is located in Texas and I believe it is the only laboratory in the country that performs this type of mold testing for the general public. Here is the contact information:

RealTime Laboratories, LLC
8325 Walnut Hill Lane Suite 125
Dallas, Texas 75231
Phone (214) 764-1160 Fax (214)890-1198
Website- www.realtimelab.com
CLIA# 45D1051736

Information on how your doctor can order these tests for you can be easily found at the website for this lab as listed above.

Also, blood IgA levels for toxic molds might have some use is determining exposure to toxic mold. This test can be ordered through any laboratory and your doctor should be able to easily order this. Salivary IgA, for toxic molds has been found in one study to correlate with exposure to toxic mold. However, I have been unable to locate a laboratory that performs this test.

Other tests that can be ordered to help in the diagnosis of toxic black mold syndrome include the following. These tests are indirect measures of toxic black mold exposure. These tests become abnormal in the body upon exposure to black mold.

MSH (Melanocyte Stimulating Hormone)
Leptin
ADH
MMP9
C3a profile
C2, C4, C4d, C3a profile
TNF
IL-I3
PAI-1
ACTH
Cortisol

Alterations in these lab values can signal a mold-toxicity problem, because the levels of these tend to be abnormal in mold-toxic individuals. This is a very new area of medicine and so many doctors may be reluctant to use tests they do not know how to interpret. Also, some of these tests may not be available at all laboratories. But some of these tests are easy to order, so give it a try and see how many your doctor is willing to order for you.

HLA testing can be used to determine your genetic type, so you can determine if you have mold susceptible genes. This information can be found on the website www.chronineurotoxins.com.

A study in 2004 showed a significant number occupants of mold-contaminated buildings tested positive for stachybotrys exposure through an ELISA test that was highly specific for macrocyclic trichothecenes. This study demonstrated that tricothecene mycotoxins can be found in some people exposed to stachybotrys through ELISA testing of the blood. I do not know of a lab that uses this method of testing and may only be available in a research setting.

In 1988, a study found that by using a monoclonal antibody, an indirect ELISA for analysis of T-2 mycotoxin could be developed. I do not believe this test is available to the general public and is only available in research situations. Hopefully in the near future, this test or other tests, will be able to be in use to determine exposure to toxic molds even at low levels.

The mycotoxins produced by molds are in a class of toxins called biotoxins. Other biotoxins in the environment are very similar to mycotoxins and act very similar to them. They are found in the venom of brown recluse spiders and the common yellowsac house spider, blue-green algaes in some fresh water lakes (cylindrospermopsis), toxic algae blooms that poison both fish and humans (red tide, Pfiesteria, ciguatera) and the toxins in Lyme disease. Biotoxins are so small and only need to be present in extremely small amounts to be toxic.

Since these biotoxins are so small, it is thought that they go undetected by our immune system. The immune system defends our bodies from foreign invaders by creating antibodies to the foreign invader. The antibody latches onto the foreign body and helps get rid of it. These antibodies are IgG, IgA, and IgM and there are specific ones of each of these types for each foreign body. In the case of biotoxins, the IgG, IgA, and IgM antibodies do not detect these small toxins. However, recently it was found that salivary IgA antibodies against molds and mycotoxins correlates well with mold exposure. Biotoxins do not create allergic symptoms in the body. Research indicates that these biotoxins act on a different system in the body called the cytokine system, which when activated, creates a lot of pain and inflammation. Pain and inflammation of different organ systems of the body can pretty much explain all the many and varied symptoms of mold toxicity. Basically the blood tests suggested to have your doctor order are substances in the body that are affected by activation of this cytokine system by mold toxins.

So, if your physician wants to order blood levels of IgG, IgA and IgM levels for the toxic molds you were exposed to, don't waste your time or your money or your blood. Most mold toxic individuals will have normal levels of these antibodies. It was concluded recently that immunologic studies of mycotoxins are not reliable nor can they be used for ruling in or out mold exposure. Also a recent court decision decided in favor of this fact as well. In fact, it is a harmful test because uneducated people will look at the results and come to the erroneous conclusion that you do not have a mold toxicity problem. That is the last thing a person with this syndrome needs.

As far as I know, this does not apply to salivary IgA levels that were shown in one study to correlate very well with mold exposure. Since only one study was done on salivary IgA against molds and mycotoxins, more studies need to be done to confirm this, so that this testing can be more widely used as a test for mold exposure.

Chapter 7
Treatment of Toxic
Black Mold Syndrome

Removal from the Source of Mold Exposure

There are several steps involved in the treatment of this condition. The first very important step in treatment of this condition is removal of yourself from the source of mold contamination.

For a majority of the population, removal of yourself from the source of mold exposure may be enough to resolve symptoms quickly and completely without any other treatment needed. This chapter is not really for those people. This group should, however, use some of the detoxification regimens to ensure that their body is free of mold toxins.

This chapter is for the minority of people, like myself, that do not get significantly better within a few weeks of avoiding exposure to toxic mold. The following treatments are helpful to speed recovery. Also, these people are not likely to get any significant improvements with any of the following treatments unless they are removed from the source of mold exposure. Some people may experience a lessening of symptoms with the following treatments, while still being exposed to mold, but most will not.

Removal of Mold Toxins from the Body

Cholestyramine Treatment:

Cholestyramine is a prescription medication that has been found clinically, to be effective in removing mold toxins from the body. It is a cholesterol-lowering medication that has been around for a long time. Its use as a cholesterol lowering medication has fallen by the wayside because of the newer cholesterol medications. It has few side effects, constipation being the most common and the most troubling. It works by binding to mold toxins that have found their way to the intestinal tract and pulling them out into the stool. Without cholestyramine, the mold toxins get reabsorbed from the gut back into the body.

The dose of cholestyramine is one packet mixed in water four times daily between meals. The package will tell you to take this medication with meals four times daily because this medication is intended to be used to lower cholesterol. So by taking the product with meals the cholestyramine will bind to all the cholesterol in the meal and prevent it from being absorbed into the body. When you take this medication between meals you allow the cholestyramine to bind to mold toxins instead of cholesterol, thus its effectiveness in toxic black mold syndrome. So take it only between meals.

Do not premix the medication ahead of time and store. It has a gritty sandy texture that is not very pleasant, but not too bad. The taste is a pleasant orange vanilla. Its medication, don't expect too much.

The length of time that one needs to take this medication probably depends on the amount and length of mold toxin exposure. Dr Shoemaker recommends a regimen of at least four weeks of full dose cholestyramine (one packet four times daily between meals). Some sources recommend that cholestyramine needs to be taken for several months.

Because cholestyramine binds to cholesterol and other fats in your intestinal tract, it will lower your cholesterol levels and also will bind to fat soluble vitamins in your intestinal tract and pull them out of your body. Over a long period of time you can develop deficiencies of the fat-soluble vitamins, vitamin A, vitamin D, and vitamin E. So, when you are on the cholestyramine, you will need to make sure you are taking a multivitamin with these vitamins in it, with your meals.

To avoid constipation, try adding fiber and extra magnesium to your diet to make your bowels more regular and loose. Magnesium supplements in the form of magnesium citrate or glycinate is best and the dose is dependent on the individual and usually ranges from 200 mg per day to 600 mg per day.

I recommend that everyone with toxic black mold syndrome take at least a four-week course of cholestyramine therapy as the first level of treatment. Then if more treatment is needed, do another month of cholestyramine or try the natural mold toxin removal methods.

Just as a side note, topically applied cholestyramine paste has been used in the treatment of spider bites especially brown recluse spider bites. My two-year-old had a very nasty looking spider bite that became very red and swollen very quickly and was the size of a baseball. I took the cholestyramine powder and mixed it with a very small amount of water to make a paste and applied it several times a day to the bite area. Within one day, we watched the redness and swelling almost completely disappear. It was absolutely amazing. It works by drawing the spider toxins out of the wound and thus stopping the whole inflammatory process. Since then I have used it successfully for bad mosquito bites. It takes the itch away immediately. It might also work for bee and wasp stings.

Natural Mold Toxin Removal:

If you are adverse to taking medications or tend to have adverse reactions to them (as a lot of people with toxic black mold syndrome do), then you may prefer the more natural means of removal of mold toxins from the body. These however are not documented to be as effective as cholestyramine. That does not mean they are not effective, just that there has not been a lot of research in this area. Theoretically, they should work, because they are purported to work for other toxins in the body.

If you have taken the cholestyramine and either are not feeling appreciably better or just want to make sure all the toxins are out, taking a course of the natural mold toxin removal remedies following the cholestyramine is a good idea. All of us could stand a little more detoxifying of toxins anyway.

Step one: Bowel Cleanse

If you are constipated, that is you do not have a bowel movement every day, you will need to get yourself more regular with supplementation. You will need to get to the point where you are having at least one, preferably 3 non-formed soft (not watery) bowel movements a day (no more than 3). You will do this with the aid of supplementation with the following.

Magnesium (magnesium glycinate, magnesium citrate, or magnesium sulfate i.e. Epsom salts).

For magnesium glycinate and magnesium citrate the dose is 200 to 1000 mg daily. The dosage of magnesium depends on the individual. Everyone is different and tolerates a different dose of magnesium. For example, for one person, a dose of 200 mg will bring on watery diarrhea while another person requires 800 mg just to bring about a loose non-formed stool.

Magnesium sulfate (Epsom salts) is a good form of magnesium. This form of magnesium is very effective and inexpensive. It has the added benefit of containing sulfate, which is a form of sulfur, which helps the body's detoxification system. Many different forms of sulfur, help the body in its detoxification, but have to be converted to sulfate first which is difficult for some people to do. The sulfur in magnesium sulfate is already converted to the sulfate form.

The dosage range for Epsom salts to be taken by mouth is 2 to 6 tsp in water (10 to 30 grams). This, by the way, tastes horrible, so you might want to explore either the other ways of getting the magnesium or the use of magnesium sulfate applied to the skin. Just as with the other types of magnesium, you will need to figure out what dose gives 1 to 3 loose unformed stools daily.

This form of magnesium can be taken also in the form of an Epsom salt bath or as a cream.

For an Epsom salt baths mix 1 to 2 cups of Epsom salts per bathtub of hot water.

For Epsom salt creams, mix 2 to 6 tsp of Epsom salts mixed with a little water and a lot of coconut oil. With this cream you get a steady dose of magnesium throughout the day.

Fiber Colon Cleanse Formula

There are many colon cleanse products on the market that contain a blend of fibers and laxative herbs to stimulate bowel movements. When using this with magnesium, it would be best to take this product once daily; and if your stool becomes too liquid, cut back on the magnesium.

Second Step: Liver Support

Once your bowels are moving regularly as they should, you can begin the second step, which is giving your body the nutritional support to help your liver do its job of detoxifying the mold toxins.

These are the supplements that boost the liver's detoxification abilities.

N-acetyl cysteine 500mg 1-2 times daily
Milk thistle 350mg daily

MSM 1000 mg 1 to 2 times daily
Lipoic acid 300 mg daily

Be careful with these supplements as they may cause your body to detoxify too rapidly and symptoms may surface. Slow down if you start getting some of the mold symptoms back. Every time I took these supplements I would get a return of the horrible toxic mold symptoms, so I had to take it really slow and gradual. So start off slow with these.

Foods like dandelion greens, radishes, beets, artichokes and green tea also help the liver detoxify.

You might want to consider getting a hair analysis done to check for mineral deficiencies. A deficiency of a mineral such as zinc or selenium could make it difficult for certain detoxification pathways in your body to run, thus blocking the detoxification process. If you are not able to do this, just taking a good quality vitamin mineral supplement every day will usually ensure you are getting all the nutrients you need.

Third Step: Mold Toxin Removal

You may start this step after you have been on the liver support supplements for a few days. There are three different remedies here. I suggest you pick the one you feel most comfortable with to try first. I would not recommend doing more than one at a time because too much detoxification is hard on your body and may even be dangerous. So with this step go slow, start gradually and stop when symptoms make you uncomfortable.

Bentonite Clay:

This works to bind toxins in the intestine and pulls them out into the stool. In this way, it works similarly to cholestyramine. However, there does not appear to be any clinical work using this supplement for mold toxin removal. Remember, there has not been much research into toxic black mold syndrome treatments because most people are still denying that it exists. So the lack of information in this area is not surprising. Without having evidence showing this supplement works for mold toxin removal, I struggled with whether or not I would include it in this book. Finally, I decided that I would include it as a possible treatment in the hopes that people with toxic mold syndrome would try it and report their results. It is a relatively harmless therapy and helps to clean out the intestines, which everyone could use a bit of. There is a risk it will cause nutrient deficiencies by pulling out nutrients as well as toxins so I recommend taking it once daily for two weeks to minimize this effect. Also I recommend taking a good multivitamin and mineral supplement every day at least four hours after the bentonite clay is consumed. It comes as a powder to mix with water or as an already-mixed slurry. It should not be taken with meals or any other supplements.

Zeolite

Zeolite is a natural mineral that is formed by volcanic eruption from the fusion of lava and ocean water. It is one of the few negatively charged minerals and has a crystalline structure that traps heavy metals and toxins. Zeolites have been used as traditional remedies in Asia for hundreds of years to promote overall health and well-being. There are many different types of zeolites but the one suggested here called clinoptilolite, is the one that has been used in animal feed and humans and has been found to be safe. Clinoptilolite is an aluminosilicate and the aluminum in this structure is so tightly bound that it would take 900 degrees Fahrenheit to split the bond. So the aluminum cannot escape into your body.

Natural zeolite has been used for years in livestock feed for animal health. On the webpage for Bear River Zeolite, it is stated that zeolite is used in the feed for dairy and beef cattle, hogs, poultry, sheep, rabbits and other animals. They claim that farms have found zeolite to eliminate animal odors and lead to greater animal health and well-being as well as longevity. As for mycotoxin binding, they state that the use of BRZ (Bear River Zeolite) and other zeolites as myco-toxin binders is not recognized by the USDA in the United States, but the effectiveness of zeolites as myco-toxin binders is recognized in many other countries. They also claim that literature and studies are pervasive in the United States.

The USFDA classifies zeolites as GRAS (generally recognized as safe) under 21 CFR Part 582.2729.

In the 1986 Chernobyl disaster, to decrease radiation poisoning from radioactive CS (a heavy metal) in cow's milk in Bulgaria, clinoptilolite was added to the cattle feed. For decontamination from radiation by radioactive CS, the children near Chernobyl were given chocolate and biscuits containing zeolite to bind and remove the radioactive heavy metal.

When zeolites are added to the feed of cows fed aflatoxin (a mycotoxin) contaminated grain, the aflatoxin in the milk was reduced. This supports the idea that zeolites remove mycotoxins from the body.

Dr. Gabriel Cousins M.D. recommends liquid zeolite to his patients for detoxification and has found it to be very successful in removing toxins. He has been using it for detoxifying women prior to becoming pregnant to lessen the amount of chemicals in the body that could harm a developing baby.

Zeolite is used as an anti-diarrhea drug in Cuba. Clinoptilolite met the standards of the Cuban Drug Quality Agency and was approved for use under the name Enterex.

A study done in 2001 and published in the *Journal of Molecular Medicine* 78 (708-720) showed zeolite to be a potential adjuvant in the treatment of cancer. They found that with zeolite in mice and dogs with tumors, there was an overall improvement in health and well-being, lifespan and decreased tumor size. In vitro studies showed zeolite induces tumor suppressor proteins and blocks cellular growth of cancer. They also did a toxicology study on mice and rats and found zeolite to be nontoxic.

After researching zeolite, I have concluded that it is safe. It comes in two forms, powdered and liquid. The liquid form is called Cellular Defense and is readily available on the Internet by a company called Waiora. Another form of liquid zeolite is called ZNatural and is made by a company called Spirit of Sunshine at www.spiritofsunshine.co.uk. It is a British company that was started by the man who developed liquid zeolite. This product is the zeolite, clinoptilolite, that has been heated to bend the molecular structure of the zeolite and then mixed in an acid solution to empty any toxins out of the molecular structure of this zeolite. Some claim that potassium is usually present in powdered zeolite and when this is removed by this purification process, a potassium deficiency may develop because zeolite binds potassium so readily and removes it from the body. One side effect of the liquid zeolite is dehydration, so it is recommended to drink plenty of water when taking it. There are a lot of testimonials to its helpfulness in a lot of diseases. Like I mentioned before, Dr. Gabriel Cousins M.D. has used liquid zeolite very successfully in his patients for detoxification.

I recommend zeolite in either form for toxic black mold syndrome mainly because I believe it works in the intestinal tract to remove mycotoxins. This would be similar to the action of cholestyramine and seaweed products (discussed in the following section).

Based on the research and toxicology studies done on animals, it appears that zeolite is not only safe, but, healthful and helpful in removing mold toxins from the body.

Sea Vegetable Products

Seaweeds have been known for their detoxification properties because they contain a certain ingredient called alginate, which acts as an intestinal detoxifier. It pulls out any toxins that circulate through the gut. You can use seaweeds, also known as sea vegetables, in your diet like arame, hijiki, nori, wakame and kombu. The seaweeds listed above are dried sea vegetables that can be found in most health food stores. They however are not as high in alginates and fucoidans as some others. They can be prepared in various dishes. Usually there are a few recipe suggestions on the package. I recommend one serving per day of one of the sea vegetable to help with detoxification. Sea vegetables are an acquired taste and many people cannot get used to the taste, so this is not for everyone. But you may only need to take them for six months to a year at the most.

A far better suggestion is to try a product called Limu Moui. The word Limu Moui basically means brown seaweed in the native language of the Kingdom of Tonga, an island in the South Pacific, where the seaweed is harvested. The Tongans have been consuming this brown seaweed for hundreds of years and attribute their excellent health to the consumption of this seaweed. Limu Moui comes in a nice tasting fruity juice drink and this is much easier to take than eating seaweed. The dosage is four ounces one to two times daily on an empty stomach. Also, this type of seaweed has a much higher content of a substance called fucoidan, which has been found to be a powerful anti-inflammatory. And as I discussed earlier, this syndrome is an inflammatory condition, thus anti-inflammatory supplements are very helpful. So with this supplement you are getting alginate a detoxifier and fucoidan, an anti-inflammatory. I have personally had tremendous results with taking this product. About nine months after leaving the contaminated office, I still had an anxious restless feeling. I just felt like I could not completely relax and sometimes I would feel shaky. After about two weeks on only four ounces a day of Limu Moui, the anxious feeling disappeared and I felt more like my normal relaxed self. And I still feel that way. I think the helpful effects on myself were due to a detoxifying effect, because even when I stopped the supplement for a few days, the good effects continued.

The two main components of this brown seaweed are fucoidan and alginate. Fucoidan has been studied extensively. There are over 650 research studies on fucoidan in the scientific literature, which can be found by searching Pubmed.org. Fucoidan is a type of carbohydrate called a complex polysaccharide. It is composed mostly of fucopyranoside and natural sulfate. It also has trace elements of galactose, xylose and glucoronic acid. Fucoidan has been shown to help with improving immune system function, relieving stomach problems, relieving allergies, improving liver function, lessening blood clotting, reduction of free radicals, reducing cholesterol levels, improvement of skin health, lowering high blood pressure, lowering blood sugar levels in diabetics, fighting cancer, fighting inflammation in the body, and removal of toxins from the body.

Alginate is another very important component of brown seaweed. Alginate, along with fucoidan too, naturally absorbs heavy metals, radioactive heavy metals, toxins and free radicals. Once bound to alginate and fucoidan these toxins do not get reabsorbed back into the body, but get excreted out into the stool. It is a perfect way to eliminate toxins from the body because it just removes them instead of having to rely on the detoxification abilities of one's body. As a holistic physician I am well aware of the fact that some people have better detoxification function than others. So a product such as this that virtually pulls toxins out of your body is very valuable.

Studies have documented this toxin binding ability of alginates in seaweeds. These studies involved the purification of alginates to be used in human tissue transplantation. The alginate naturally binds to endotoxins and other toxins in the environment and these toxins have to be removed by a special purification process, so they can be used in the transplantation of cells.

Therefore, they have indirectly shown that alginates bind to endotoxins, which are natural organic toxins. Mycotoxins are also natural organic toxins so they should also bind to alginates.

The testimonials on this brown seaweed (Limu Moui) are amazing. To me, I think they have to be due to removal of toxins because they are more dramatic than any other nutritional product I have ever seen. Although they do not demonstrate that this product is a black mold treatment, here are a few testimonials that I know personally and think are pretty amazing.

A patient of mine introduced me to Limu Moui in February of 2006. She had such an amazing recovery from chronic fatigue and fibromyalgia that she attributed to Limu Moui that I had to check it out. After 2 months of taking Limu Moui, her fatigue and fibromyalgia had disappeared. She had bloodwork done by me both before she started taking Limu and 2 months after, which were amazing. Before taking Limu her female hormones and DHEA were low for a woman in her mid-forties. Also her antibodies against her thyroid were very high meaning her Hashimotos Thyroiditis was very active. After 2 months on the Limu, her female hormones and DHEA were elevated to that of a healthy woman. DHEA, which I consider to be a marker for general overall health had shot up to a healthy level at the upper limit of normal! That really impressed me. Also her thyroid antibodies dropped much lower, suggesting her Hashimotos Thyoiditis was not as active. Now over one year later, she still takes Limu Moui, still has tons of energy, and has no fibromyalgia pain. She says the amount of time she spent sleeping when she was sick is now the amount of time she spends awake. We do not know what caused her fatigue and fibromyalgia. Could it have been an unknown exposure to mycotoxins in her environment? I think it's possible. Or perhaps she had a build up of another toxin that her body could not eliminate without help. She continues to take the limu and continues to feel great. There are clues that suggest to me that the greatest action of the limu in this patient was toxin removal. One is that she says she can now stop the limu and still feel good. The other is that she describes a slow gradual improvement over months and continual improvement the longer she continues on it. That really suggests detoxification to me.

My mother-in-law started taking it for just general health improvement. She said she felt great before she started it. Then one week after starting the Limu, she said the tinnitis (ringing in her ears) went away. Then 2 weeks later she reported her neck didn't hurt as much. It's amazing how you don't realize what symptoms you are having until they are gone.

Yet another sea vegetable product to try is called Modifilan, which is, also, brown seaweed, only in a dry encapsulated form. It is also rich in detoxifying alginates and anti-inflammatory fucoidans. It is made by a company called Pacific Standard Distributors, Inc. and can be obtained off the website www.modifilan.com. The dosage is three capsules in the morning on an empty stomach for one week then gradually increase to six capsules daily in the morning on an empty stomach for four months.

With any of the above therapies, just keep in mind that it will take some time to remove the toxins from your body. Because these therapies work in the intestinal tract to pull out the toxins, it just takes time. It took me six months to feel better doing some of the above therapies. But because I was researching treatments for this on my own, I did not have all the information on different therapies right away. So, some of these treatments I did not try or even know about until several months after leaving the mold contaminated office. One of the most important things to do is to stop your exposure to toxic black mold.

Far Infrared Saunas

Another way to detoxify is through the use of saunas. I did not use this form of detoxification because it was not available to me. Traditional steam saunas are also effective though not as comfortable due to the hot steam that many people find uncomfortable. Far infrared saunas use far infrared heaters to warm the skin and not the air. They are used to warm babies in hospital nurseries. Not only are they more effective at detoxifying because the heat goes deeper into the skin, but they are also much more comfortable because they do not heat the air. According to studies, the sweat induced by a conventional sauna was found to be 95 to 97% water whereas the sweat induced by a far infrared sauna was found to be 80 to 85% water and the other parts were cholesterol, fat soluble toxins, toxic heavy metals, sulfuric acid, sodium, ammonia and uric acid. This high concentration of toxins and heavy metals was not found in the sweat induced by conventional saunas.

Saunas are to be used with caution and their use should be discussed with your doctor first.

If your doctor gives approval for sauna use, then you still should proceed slowly and carefully, because, as saunas remove toxins, you can have a return or worsening of your symptoms.

Be aware that if you are on medications that should stay at a constant level such as insulin or seizure medications, these medicine levels can drop due to the increased detoxifying process that is going on. This could cause problems.

Because a sauna will cause a release of toxins from the fat cells into the bloodstream, a person with mold toxicity should proceed very slowly to avoid the uncomfortable symptoms caused by mold toxins. Basically, if you go too fast you might relive the mold toxicity experience. I discovered this in myself when exercising. Within twenty minutes of breaking a sweat, I would experience a panic attack and the horrible sensation that I was going to pass out. It made working out impossible for me until my body became less toxic.

Also, if you had ever used recreational drugs, a sauna may cause you to relive those experiences as you detoxify out these drugs.

ALWAYS START SLOW! Start using the sauna at 100 F, in short five to ten minute sessions at first. Some people may only be able to tolerate one minute at first. You need to build up a tolerance. If you are having trouble tolerating the heat, start with a lower temperature.

After the first few saunas check the blood pressure, temperature, respiratory rate, weight and pulse rate. People who are very ill should have these checked every ten to fifteen minutes, while in the sauna.

General Rules:

If your BP, pulse or respiratory rate increase by 10 points while in the sauna, get out of the sauna for the day.

Also, if your oral temperature goes over 100 F while in the sauna...GET OUT!

STOP when you experience headache, nausea, fast heart rate, weakness, irregular heart rate, shortness of breath, dizziness, disorientation, muscle cramps, muscle spasms, muscle twitching, or any adverse symptom.

If you weigh less after a sauna, you did not drink enough water to make up for the loss.

Weigh your towels before and after the sauna and then drink the difference in weight in purified water.

Keep a diary of your symptoms

The usual range of temperatures to set the sauna at range from 100 F or less to 140 F. Some people may never go over 120 F.

If at any time you feel uncomfortable, STOP, or open the door, towel off and cool down.

While in the sauna, keep wiping off the sweat with a clean dry towel.

Shower in lukewarm water as soon as possible after a sauna to prevent toxins from being reabsorbed.

If you can not do more than fifteen minutes at a time you can do short fifteen minute sessions two to four times a day.

Know that the symptoms of heat stroke are dry and/or cold skin.

Magnesium is the main mineral to be lost in the greatest amount in the sweat.

Any mineral deficiency you have going into the sauna will be accentuated with the losses through the sweat in the sauna.

The average American diet is deficient in magnesium, providing only 40% of the magnesium needed.

Zinc and calcium are the second most commonly lost minerals in the use of saunas.

Supplements necessary to take prior to a sauna:

1. Drink at least 1-2 quarts of purified water for each hour of a sauna.
2. Magnesium glycinate or magnesium citrate 300 mg for each hour of a sweat.
3. Calcium citrate 500 mg for each hour of sweating.
4. zinc citrate 25mg for each hour of sweating
5. one tsp Trisalts for each hour of sweating.

Supplements to take following the sauna:

1. A general digestive enzyme supplement.
2. Buffered Vitamin C (3000 mg of Vitamin C).
3. Lipoic acid 300 mg
4. N-Acetyl Cysteine 500mg
5 Milk Thistle 350mg
6. 2 large glasses of purified water.

Exercise

Exercise works similar to a sauna to remove toxins by sweating them out. Exercise also has the added benefit of getting your lymphatic system moving to help move the toxins out of the body. Try to exercise as much as you can while detoxifying from black mold to help move the toxins out of your system. I could not exercise when my body was really toxic because every time I tried to, I would almost pass out as soon as I broke a sweat and toxins were released into my bloodstream. So, do as much as you can every day, but be careful not to overdo it as it may result in a dramatic return of symptoms.

Symptom Relief:

While you are going through all this detoxification, it's helpful to have some relief from the symptoms. Here are some suggestions for supplements and diet that help to lessen inflammation and thus relieve symptoms in toxic black mold syndrome.

Supplements:

These are both oils that decrease inflammation in the body:
Flaxseed oil 1 tbsp daily
Fish oil (420mg EPA and 300mg DHA per capsule) 3 daily.

These help relieve any allergy components of toxic mold syndrome:
Natural antihistamines (Aller-max by Country Life or Natural D-Hist by Orthomolecular)
Apples and onions are natural antihistamines because they are loaded with quercetin.

Natural anti-inflammatory supplements:
Quercetin 300 mg one to 3 times daily
MSM or sulfer 1000mg 2 to 3 times daily
Coenzyme Q-10 100mg 1 to 3 times daily
Limu Moui 4oz 1 – 2 times daily

For some reason an amylose free diet helps relieve the symptoms of toxic mold syndrome and amylase supplements seem to help relieve the allergy component of this syndrome as well.
Amylase supplements in capsule form. Amylase is an enzyme that digests the sugar amylose.
The amylose free diet (avoid bananas, potatoes, sugar and all grains except corn)

Anti-Inflammatory Diet Suggestions:

These same suggestions can be found in the elimination and healing diets later in this chapter. The purpose of the following list is to explain that certain dietary suggestions are specifically to reduce inflammation and remove toxins from the body.

Avoid red meat, high fat dairy, and pork, shellfish

These foods have saturated fats that promote inflammatory mediators in the body.

Eat plenty of fish

Fish has a lot of EPA and DHA that the body uses to produce anti-inflammatory mediators. Be careful to avoid those fish that are more likely to contain biotoxins from a certain type of algae. See the diets at the end of this chapter for the specific fish to avoid.

Raw unheated honey

This contains loads of enzymes, especially amylase which helps with allergies

Omega 3 eggs

These are loaded with DHA, which produces anti-inflammatory mediators.

Nuts and seeds

These contain good oils that the body uses to make anti-inflammatory mediators in the body.

Low fat dairy products

These are acceptable...nonfat would be best because the saturated fat in full fat dairy products promote inflammation.

Beans

These contain a lot of minerals and are an alternate source of protein other than fish and eggs.

Raw vegetables

These contain enzymes and alkalinize the body, which decreases inflammation.

Raw fruits

These contain a lot of enzymes and they also alkalinize the body, which decreases inflammation.

Avocados

Avocados have a lot of good fats as well as a lot of lipase to digest the fat. This raw fat seems to really help the body remove toxins from fat cells.

Raw coconuts

Raw coconut also contains a lot of fat and lipase and helps remove toxins.

Olive oil
Coconut oil

These are good oils that don't promote inflammation, and coconut oil has lauric acid, which has anti-fungal properties.

Sea vegetables

These have detoxification properties because they contain alginate, a detoxifying substance.

Miso soup

Miso soup is loaded with enzymes and is known to have detoxification properties

Antifungal Treatment:

There are many options for antifungal treatment both naturally and with drugs, but they all should include probiotic supplementation to keep good bacteria in the intestinal tract to compete against any fungal or yeast overgrowth.

Probiotic supplementation:

I recommend a high quality high potency probiotic to be taken continuously throughout recovery from toxic black mold syndrome.

I recommend buying a brand that needs refrigeration, as I believe those types are more potent. These probiotics should be taken at least once a day, preferably two hours apart from any antifungal supplements. The ones I recommend are made by Natren.

Lactobacillus acidophilus super strain DDS 2 billion cfu - ½ tsp 1 to 2 x daily

Bifidobacterium bifidum Super strain Malyoth 2 billion cfu ½ tsp 1 to 2 x daily

Bifidobacterium infantis Super strain NLS 1 billion cfu ¼ tsp 1 to 2 x daily

Lactobacillus Bulgaricus super strain LB-51 2 billion cfu ½ tsp 1 to 2 x daily

Antifungal treatments:

Then the antifungal choices are as follows:

Natural Supplements: These can be found over the counter in most health food stores.

Oregano oil extract 10 drops 3 times daily
Candicid Forte by Orthomolecular 2caps 3 times daily
Three-lac by Global Health Trax 1 to 4 packets daily for 1 to 2 months then one packet daily.

Medications: These have to be prescribed by your doctor and include the following:

Nystatin oral powder
Diflucan
Sporonox
Lamisil

Basic Supplementation Program for Toxic Black Mold Syndrome:

In addition to the other supplements recommended throughout this book, here is a list of basic ones that should not be missed in order for your system to function optimally and have all the nutrients required to detoxify the mold toxins.

Take a good quality multivitamin mineral; one that either contains the following nutrients or, if it does not, then a multivitamin and mineral supplement with nutrients added to equal the following:

Vitamin D 1000 IU daily
Vitamin E with alpha and gamma tocopherols 400 IU daily
Zinc 30 mg daily
Selenium 200 mcg daily
Vitamin B12 1000 to 2000 mcg daily
Vitamin C 3000 mg daily

Antifungal/Low Mycotoxin Diet:

The diet I recommend for treatment of Toxic Mold Syndrome accomplishes three things.

First of all, it is a low carbohydrate diet that essentially starves out any fungus that may have set up camp in your body, most likely in the intestinal tract or sinus cavities. With Toxic Mold Syndrome this is likely for a number of reasons. One, being, that mycotoxins in and of themselves suppress the immune system, making it more likely for fungal growth to occur. Another reason is that some of the spores that were breathed in during toxic mold exposure might have set up camp somewhere in the body most likely in the intestines or the sinus cavities. Finally, with toxic mold syndrome the immune system is suppressed, and oftentimes bacterial or viral infections set in and the person inevitably gets put on an antibiotic. The antibiotic kills off the good bacteria in the intestinal tract, and candida, which normally inhabits the intestines or another fungus, perhaps the one you have been breathing in, starts to overgrow. Remember the spores that are breathed into the lungs are dormant molds looking for a place to grow. So it is quite possible that a fungus can grow in your body. I know for a fact this to be true because as a physician I saw a lot of stool samples on patients come back showing candida growth and other fungal growth in the intestines as well.

The second thing that this diet accomplishes is elimination of mycotoxin containing foods. If you have Toxic Mold Syndrome your body is already flooded with mycotoxins. You essentially don't need any more. And the lessened load of mycotoxins will free up your body's detoxification mechanisms and allow the mycotoxins you have already accumulated through the toxic mold exposure to be excreted as quickly as possible.

The third thing this diet accomplishes is a reduction of foods that contribute to inflammation in the body as discussed in the previous section titled symptom relief.

The diet I recommend is an adaptation of diets recommended by others. It is adapted from Dr. William Crook's anti-candida diet, Dr. Shoemaker's amylose free diet and Doug Kaughman's 3 phase, antifungal diet plan. It is similar to the anti-candida diet I have been recommending to my patients for the past ten years. It is also based on personal experience with toxic mold syndrome and what helped me, and others that I knew with the syndrome. It also incorporates some other principles I believe to be important, namely that raw foods are healing. There are two different phases of the diet. The first phase is the elimination phase. The second phase is the healing phase.

The Mycotoxin and Fungus Elimination Phase of the Diet

This phase limits mycotoxins as much as possible. It is also the lowest carbohydrate part of the diet program. It is because of these restrictions that it is also the hardest part of the diet! I recommend doing it for the first month along with cholestyramine. Then I recommend continuing another month on the elimination phase, along with an antifungal supplement or antifungal drug. It helps, on this diet, to eat a lot of avocados and coconuts because their high beneficial fat content helps to keep you full and not feeling starving all the time. Feeling hungry is a common complaint of this diet because of the low carbohydrate content. The types of fat in avocados and coconuts are very healthful and beneficial. The diet recommendations are as follows.

MYCOTOXIN AND FUNGUS ELIMINATION PHASE

ALLOWABLE FOOD	FOODS TO AVOID

FRUITS:#

lemons limes	bananas
grapefruits	pineapples
Green apples	melons
blueberries	grapes
strawberries	oranges
raspberries	pears
berries	peaches
	dried fruits

VEGETABLES:#

lettuce, green beans	corn, potatoes,
tomatoes, broccoli, peas,	sweet potatoes
eggplant, peppers, onions,	dried beans
garlic, squash,	peas
brussel sprouts, cauliflower	turnips
cabbage, collard greens,	rutabagas
kale, dandelion greens,	beets
celery, mustard greens,	
turnip greens, artichokes,	
asparagus, parsley, cilantro	
Jicama, leeks, scallions, radishes,	
zucchini, cucumbers,	
**RAW AVOCADOS	

GRAINS:

none	rice, corn,
	wheat, rye
	oats

NUTS/SEEDS:

raw soaked walnuts, almonds cashews,
pumpkin seeds soaked and dried pistachios
sesame seeds peanuts
sunflower seeds (soaked and dried)
nut butters
**RAW COCONUT

OILS:

olive oil	corn oil
coconut oil	peanut oil
sesame oil	margarine
flaxseed oil	

DAIRY:

yogurt (unsweetened) low fat	milk
kefir (unsweetened) low fat	aged cheeses
goat cheese	ice cream
cottage cheese low fat	blue cheese
sour cream low fat	whipped cream
cream cheese low fat	
butter small amounts	
eggs (high DHA type)	

BEVERAGES:

fresh squeezed lemonade or limeade	Coffee, tea, soda
Seltzer water, filtered water	alcohol, beer
Herb teas	Fruit juice
wine	

YEAST PRODUCTS:

none	bread, beer
	Mushrooms
	pastries

FISH:

salmon, cod, haddock	***mackeral,
Tilapia	skipjack tuna
Sushi##	yellowtail
Albacore and yellowfin tuna	ocean perch

MEATS:

Chicken and turkey###	breaded meats
Lamb	pork
beef (preferably on the rare side)	sausage
	smoked meats

VINEGARS AND PICKLED FOODS:

unpasturized apple	pickles, green
cider vinegar, black	olives, soy
olives not preserved	sauce
in vinegar	

SWEETENERS:

stevia,	sugar,
	high fructose
	corn syrup
	maple syrup
	honey
	aspartame
	saccharin
	Splenda

Nuts should be raw (uncooked) and should be soaked in water in the refrigerator for about 8 to 12 hours and then dried in a food dehydrator at 104 degrees or in an oven set to 100 if you have that option.

** Raw coconut and raw avocados are raw fats that are especially good at helping the body to detoxify. They do this by replacing the body fat containing toxins with new fat. And the benefit of raw fats is that they contain all the fat digesting enzymes because they are raw, so your body utilizes them well. Raw foods contain enzymes that your body uses to help digest the food. I found these foods to be very helpful in reducing symptoms of mold toxicity, and they also seemed to relieve anxiety.

***Certain seafood is more likely to be contaminated with certain toxins in the ocean from toxic algae. These fish are more likely to be affected and would best be avoided if you are susceptible to mold toxins.

vegetables and fruits should not have mold on them or large blemishes

##Sushi is raw fish so it contains raw fat. Raw fat is helpful to remove mold toxins from the body. Make sure you buy sushi from a reputable sushi bar to avoid food poisoning.

###Ideally meats and dairy should be from grass-fed animals rather than grain-fed, but if that's not possible or too difficult to find (which is usually the case) then try to get meat or dairy not given hormones or antibiotics. Beef should be eaten on the rare side to get some raw fats. I don't suggest eating poultry or lamb rare. Limit the consumption of beef and lamb because of the inflammation that red meat tends to cause in the body.

THE HEALING PHASE OF THE DIET

FOODS TO EAT	FOODS TO AVOID

FRUITS:#

Lemons, limes	bananas
Grapefruits, oranges	cantaloupe
Strawberries	dried fruits
Blueberries, raspberries	
Grapes, pineapples	
Peaches, pears, apples	
Watermelons,	

VEGETABLES:#

Lettuce, green beans	potatoes,
Tomatoes, broccoli, peas	sweet potatoes
Eggplant, peppers, onions	turnips
Garlic, squash, cabbage	rutabagas
Brussel sprouts, cauliflower	beets
Collard greens, kale, dandelion	
Greens, celery, mustard greens,	
Turnip greens, artichokes,	
Asparagus, parsley, cilantro,	
Jicama, leeks, scallions, corn	
Radishes, zucchini, cucumbers	
dried beans or peas	
**RAW AVOCADOS	

GRAINS:

brown rice	wheat, oats, rye
	corn

NUTS/SEEDS:

Raw soaked walnuts or almonds
Pumpkin seed soaked and dried
Sesame seeds soaked and dried
Sunflower seeds soaked and dried
Nut butters
**RAW COCONUTS (mature or young)

cashews
pistachios
peanuts

OILS:

Olive oil
Coconut oil
Sesame oil
Flaxseed oil

corn oil
peanut oil
margarine

DAIRY:

Yogurt (unsweetened) low fat
Kefir (unsweetened) low fat
Goat cheese
Milk low fat
Cottage cheese low fat
Cream cheese low fat
Sour cream (low fat)
Butter small amounts
Eggs (high DHA type)

aged cheese
blue cheese
ice cream
whipped cream

BEVERAGES:

Fresh squeezed lemonade or limeade
Seltzer water, filtered water, herb teas
Fresh squeezed fruit or vegetable juice

coffee, tea
sodas, alcohol
beer, wine,
Fruit juices

YEAST:
None

bread
Pastries
Mushrooms

FISH:

Salmon, cod , haddock	***mackeral
Tilapia, sole	skipjack tuna
Sushi ##	yellow tail
Albacore and yellowfin tuna	ocean perch
Sardines	shellfish

MEATS:

Chicken or turkey###	pork
Lamb	breaded meats
Beef (preferably on the rare side)	sausage
	smoked meats

VINEGARS AND PICKLED FOODS:

Un-pasteurized apple cider vinegar	pickles
Black olives not preserved in vinegar	green olives
	Soy sauce

SWEETENERS:

Stevia	sugar
####Raw unheated honey	high fructose corn syrup
	maple syrup
	heated honey
	aspartame
	saccharin
	Splenda

#freshly juiced greens especially parsley with carrots and fruit helps the body detoxify mold toxins. I found too much would bring back symptoms of mold toxicity.

raw honey contains many enzymes especially amylase which is helpful with allergies and seems to help relieve symptoms of mold toxicity.

71

Chapter 8
How to Test Your House
for Toxic Black Mold

For a professional mold inspection of your home call the National Association of Mold Professionals to get a referral to a mold inspector in your area. In my experience, this was a very expensive way to go, and I don't believe a lot of people will be able to afford it. At the time, I was sick and desperate, so I chose to have it professionally done. Now in hindsight, I wish I had done it myself because I am still digging out of the financial nightmare incurred by mold testing and remediation. I wish I had known how to do it myself back then. But if you can afford it, having someone else do all the dirty work is much easier especially if you are sick.

I know there are a lot of people out there who are absolutely terrified of the financial nightmare of mold remediation and would rather suffer than have to go into thousands of dollars of debt. I know these people may also try to remove the mold themselves without any advice at all. For those people I recommend they do it all on their own but safely for a fraction of the cost were they to have someone else do it. I believe part of the problem this country faces right now with this mold problem is that it is all too costly for the average person to do, so they end up doing nothing and continuing to live and be sick in their moldy environment. I think we need to empower the people in our country to stand up and take matters into their own hands and clean up their environment safely. This chapter is all about how to test your home without going bankrupt. This is based on my personal experience watching mold professionals in my home.

First do a nonprofessional inspection of your home or workplace. Follow the following steps to do this.

1. Do the sniff test in all rooms of the building.

Before you do this, spend some time outdoors for 1 to 2 hours so you are not accustomed to the odor in your house. It's amazing what odors some people cannot even smell anymore in their own homes.

Do you smell a musty, moldy or urine-like smell in any room? Does your basement smell moldy or musty? Open cupboards and cabinets and get a good whiff. This is a very accurate way to find mold if you have a good nose. If you don't have a good nose or have a cold or sinus problems all the time, then have a friend who does not live with you do this test for you. My friend, Janet, told me my basement smelled very musty and moldy, and I could not even smell that after being exposed to it so much. Mark on a piece of paper all the rooms that have an odor.

2. Then go throughout your house and do a visual inspection of the musty-smelling rooms and make a note of any questionable areas.

Mold can be brown, black, green or white.

Aspergillus and penicillium species can grow on cement walls and floors, fiberglass insulation, carpets, shower tiles etc and can live off just the humidity in the air if it's above 55%. So these molds do not have to have a leak or a water source to live.

Stachybotrys and chaetomium, on the other hand, cannot live off the humidity in the air and need a definite continuous source of water to live, such as a leaky roof or pipe. These molds live on cellulose, wallboard; paper, wood, and cotton. And, as I have stated before, these molds are the most detrimental to human health.

3. Find the water. A mold inspector uses a piece of equipment called a hygrometer, which detects moisture. You can purchase one of these for $295 from Professional Equipment.com. You can then take your hygrometer and test all the questionable areas of your house. Make sure you check bathroom tiles around your tub, as this is a common area for moisture to collect. The cost of a professional mold inspection of your house may run about $250, so it may be worth it having a mold inspector come out and do all the work. However, if you are pretty sure where the mold is, then you might not even need the hygrometer to find the problem. If that is the case, you can just skip on to the next section on testing for mold. If you are going to purchase a hygrometer, then you should know that they are easy to use. You can hold them up to any surface and determine if there is moisture or water behind it. It's like being able to see inside your walls.

Make a note of all the areas with high moisture readings.

Okay, so now you should have a better idea of the mold status of your house. You should have one or more potential problem areas.

The next step is to test for mold.

Testing for Mold

Swab sample:

If you have visible mold growth, this test is an option and is a much cheaper way to go. First, wear the respirator that you are going to need any way if you are going to be doing the mold removal yourself. It is essential to protect your lungs from flying spores as you disturb the mold. Also wear plastic or leather gloves to protect your hands and do not have any skin exposed (no shorts, wear long pants and a long sleeved shirt. This is to protect your skin from mold spores. The toxins from mold spores can be absorbed right through your skin and can also cause a rash in the area exposed to the spores. This is especially true with stachybotrys. Then, make sure that the mold will come off when swabbed with a Q-tip. Then buy a Prolab Mold Test kit from the Home Depot for 10.00 and follow the directions for getting a swab sample of mold. Analysis of the sample by Prolab costs about 30.00 and takes almost a month to come back. I think the swab test in this kit works well but I do not think the air test done with this kit is very accurate at all. I did both the Prolab air test with the Petri dish and the air sampling with the spore trap simultaneously on the first floor of my house. The home depot test showed low levels of cladosporin while the air spore trap test showed very high levels of aspergillus/penicillium species. These were totally different results for the same general area. The air-sampling test was of course more accurate.

Air Sampling:

I think this is a much better way to go because you are actually testing what you are breathing in the air. This test definitely is the only way to go if you can smell a musty moldy odor in your house but cannot find the source. The mold source could be in the walls or in the air ducts.

With this test you can determine what kind of mold is present and how many spores are present (which indicates the extent of the problem).

This test is performed by pumping air through a container called a spore trap, at 5 liters per minute. The spore trap catches both viable (living) and nonviable (dead) spores. Some sources suggest only a viable spore sample is the best, but other sources claim both viable and nonviable are needed because dead spores are just as toxic as live ones. I agree with the latter, and nonviable spore trapping is much less expensive too.

Air sampling is the testing that a mold inspector will do and will most likely charge anywhere form 600 to 1000 dollars for. It cost me $600 to test my house and that included testing only two rooms and the outside. An outside sample is always needed for comparison of normal molds in the surrounding environment.

There are a few different types of air sampling tests, but the type I had purchased was the EMS micro5 Basic (Indoor Air Quality) IAQ kit with megalite pump from Professional Equipment.com. The cost is about 329.95 plus shipping and handling. This cost includes 10 cassettes to collect the samples in.

You will need to do an air sample in each room you suspect mold and then one outdoors to determine the level of outdoor mold that may be affecting your indoor sample. You should do the sample with the house closed up for the preceding twenty-four hours. Keep the windows shut. If you have a forced air system with air ducts, you will want to do one sample with the air ducts on and one with the air ducts off to determine if there is mold in the air ducts. Set the air sampler in the middle of each room about two to three feet off the ground. If you are using the Micro5 IAQ with megalite pump, you need to hook the clear hose from the air pump to the micro5 cassette and set the pump to 5 liters per minute and set a timer to five minutes as you turn on the pump. Once five minutes is up turn off the pump and disconnect the hose from the cassette. Mark on the cassette the date and time the sample was taken and the room in which the sample was taken. That's it! There are directions that come with the sampler but they are not that good. I had to call the company EMS to get directions. When finished with the sampling, you will have a bunch of cassettes that need to be sent to a lab for analysis. I used a lab called:

IMS Laboratory
3250 Old Farm Lane, Suite 1
Walled Lake, MI 48390
www.imslaboratory.com
(877) 665-3373
(248) 669-1412 fax

This is not a viable (live) sample so you don't have to rush it to a lab. It takes just a few days for the lab to analyze this (include shipping times if you do not have a lab that will do this locally).

To have your samples analyzed at this lab runs around $21.00 per sample for each room. We are still under $600.00. Now, when you consider that you will need before mold removal and after mold removal samples, that's where the savings come in. If you have both home and work that needs to be checked, this would save you a lot of money. You can also test more rooms in your house than just two. And finally, you have the equipment for future use if you were to move and need to check a new house before you buy it. If you are a toxic black mold syndrome victim, you will always have to careful of where you live and work. That is why I bought this kit. I don't want to go through what I went through again and I want to have the ability to test any new home or workplace.

And, I no longer just blindly trust building owners to do the right thing, and maintain their building properly.

The other option is to purchase a kit called the ExaminAir Home Test Kit, www.examinair.net. This test uses the same IAQ air sampling that professional mold inspectors use. It can be ordered by contacting My Healthy Home at (866) 743-8563 or by ordering off their website at www.myhealthyhome.info. It is made for use by the general public, so it is much more user friendly than buying your own air sampling equipment. It tests for molds and other allergens such as dust and dust mites. The cost is $400 per kit and that will test three rooms plus an outdoor sample. Analysis is included in the cost of the kit as well as shipping. If you want personalized expert advice regarding your results, the cost will be an additional $40.00.

If you are waiting for the Prolab (home depot) analysis to come back, you have a whole month to wait. If you are able to spend time away from your house, do as much of this as possible. Go away for the weekend or take a week vacation time. Or stay with family or friends if that option exists for you. The point is, stop your exposure to the mold that is making you sick. You may not feel better right away after leaving, but you might. As I stated before some people get better sooner than others because they detoxify better. If it is the summertime and the weather is nice, camp out in a tent in your own backyard. Or if you have a screen porch, camp out there. At the very least, if it's summer, leave all your windows open all the time with fans on to keep the air circulating.

If your testing comes back showing toxic mold spores are present then you have a problem. You may be wondering how you are going to interpret the results. This should help you.

First, you should compare the indoor samples to the outdoor sample. If any mold is higher indoors than outdoors you may have a problem.

If any stachybotrys or chaetomium spores at all are found indoors, even if it's just one, you have a problem. At my workplace we found 9000 spores per cubic meter of stachybotrys and 4000 of chaetomium. Those are pretty hefty amounts. Even amounts in the hundreds could be harmful.

If any aspergillus or penicillium species are found, then you have a problem. This is a toxic mold, but it is easier to fix because most of the time it lives on the humidity in the air, so a dehumidifier can greatly improve the problem. The bad ones are stachybotrys and chaetomium and any levels of those are considered to be harmful.

Chapter 9
If You Have Toxic Black Mold, How Do You Fix It?

Remediation is the term the industry uses to describe cleaning up a mold problem and fixing any water leaks so the problem does not reoccur. This usually requires ripping out wallboard and fixing leaky roofs or pipes as well as removal of any moldy material like wallboard, insulation, wood or carpeting. I watched most of it being done in my house, and it's not rocket science. It requires some muscle and lots of protection against mold spores. If you are sick, you may not be up to the task yourself. I know that I wasn't when it happened to me. I was too sick to don a respirator and go down to the basement and rip out insulation. It's not a good idea to put on a respirator if you are feeling short of breath as I was.

So your options are to hire a mold remediation company or have another less sick member of your family or an outside handyman do the work. A mold remediation company is definitely your best bet if you can afford it. The company I used was:

Mold Experts of Michigan
3549 Airport Rd., Suite 104
Waterford, MI 48329
1-888-950 MOLD (6653)
www.moldexpertsofmichigan.com

They were very professional and quick. It was easy and they took care of the vapor barriers and filters. The end result for me was a clean mold free basement in a short period of about a week and a half. For a recommendation of a mold remediation company near you call National Association of Mold Professionals (NAMP) at (248) 669-5673 or go to their website at www.moldpro.org.

In the case of a family member or a handyman you will have to provide them with the proper safety equipment, which is a respirator with frequent filter changes and a suit and gloves to protect the skin. A handyman should be able to do the job at a much lower cost..I had part of my work done by a handyman at a much lower cost. However, their level of care in not contaminating the rest of your house is not as high as a professional mold remediation company. So that part will be up to you, which I will explain as we go along.

Step 1. First, pick a room to remediate if you have more than one. Then you will need to remove from the room things you want to clean and keep clean. If your house is contaminated with spores, those spores are on everything, and you will have to wash everything or throw it out. Standard practice had previously been to toss everything out that had been contaminated with stachybotrys spores, but now it is suggested to just wash any contaminated items with bleach. With clothing and blanketing you can use detergent plus 20 Mule Team Borax with each load to kill spores.

Take everything outside or into your garage (never the basement) I put everything in my garage and a big screened in tent outside in my backyard. In retrospect, I would not recommend the screen-tent as things will get a little wet.

Step 2: Next, you will have to put up what they call a vapor barrier which is basically a sheet of plastic taped up tight around a door, preferably with a zippered door to make it easier to get in and out. But, I found it is hard to find the zippered door vapor barriers, so the next best option would be to just tape up plastic with duct tape to cover the door. This is to protect the rest of the house from being contaminated with mold spores. Sheets of plastic can be found at any home improvement store.

Step 3: Rent a commercial high powered HEPA filter from either a mold remediation company or a rental store and put it into the sealed off room. This will create a negative air pressure in the room to keep the spores in the room and not flying all over your house. I rented mine from a mold remediation company for about $400 for a week. Run it continuously in that room until the next day or until the day after you finish the room.

Step 4: Put on your protective suit and respirator. Make sure the filter in the respirator is in place and clean. The respirator I purchased was the 3M Mold Remediation Respirator Kit 67097 and can be purchased from Professional equipment.com at 129.95, which includes two filters. It comes in different sizes and covers the whole face to protect the eyes too. The disposable protective suit can also be purchased from professional equipment for 7.95 each. The suit is not a necessity, as you can just wear a long sleeved shirt and pants. Just make sure you remove them and wash them in detergent and 20 mule team Borax when you are done.

Step 5: It's Demolition time. This can be the fun part if you are into this sort of thing. Remove any wallboard, carpeting, cabinets, etc. with obvious mold growth present. If you cannot see mold, but the room tested high for spores, it's probably in the carpet or behind the walls or in the ceiling. Removal of the carpet usually reveals mold on the wood underneath or on the carpet backing. If you suspect it may be behind walls, start with one wall first. If you are knocking down walls you should turn off the electricity in your house. If you are working in the bathroom or kitchen you should turn off the water too. It's probably a good idea to turn off both water and electric at demolition time. Remember, if this is too much for you, a handyman or building contractor would be ideal. But, you should do all the proper work like the vapor barrier and the commercial HEPA filter. But if you are not wearing a respirator you should not be in the house while this work is being done. Even when the day is over, it would be better if you were not in the house because more than likely there are some mold spores that escaped the room. Camp outside or at the very least leave all the windows open if it's warm.

Step 6: Look for leaking pipes. Look for leaks coming from the roof. Are there areas behind the walls that are wet? If so, you will need to find out where the water is coming from. Sometimes the problem may be too difficult to fix without professional help, and you should have an idea of this by now for this particular room at least. You might have to hire a plumber to fix a leaky pipe or have your roof inspected for leaks. A roofing company will usually do an inspection and estimate for free. Most people will not take on roofing their own house, so that is something you will have to have done, if need be. It is important to fix all sources of water intrusion in your house or the mold will just grow back. If you cannot find the source of water intrusion, you will have to hire someone to do this.

Step 7: Wash down any cement floors or walls with bleach to kill any mold.

Step 8: Replacement of the moldy stuff. This is not completely necessary if you don't mind living with a torn up house for a while until funds get better. It is certainly better than living in a moldy house. Wood that is moldy should be replaced, but you will have to make sure you are not tearing out any load bearing walls. You will probably have to hire a building contractor to determine that, if you do not know.

Step 9: Repeat the above steps for all the suspicious rooms in your house.

Step 10: Leave the HEPA filter on for a few days after you are done with the whole house.

Step 11: Retest the whole house with the air sampler one week later.

If it is your unfinished basement that has mold growth on the cement walls and floors, wash off the mold with bleach and then run a dehumidifier continuously to keep the humidity below 55%. A low humidity will prevent the type of mold that grows on cement from growing back.

Be careful with the application of any biocidal or antifungal agents, as it is believed and shown in studies that use of these agents creates resistant strains of fungus with more toxic spores. One study in 2003 showed that the use of a biocide in plasterboard did not limit the mold growth and increased the cytotoxic potential of the spores. So when treated with things that inhibit mold growth, the mold retaliates by putting out spores that are more toxic. This is probably a defense mechanism. More toxic algaes are thought to result from widespread use of algaecides in lakes and ponds. Toxic algae in the ocean is thought to be caused by damage to reefs that algae live on and a resultant increase in toxin production in response to this.

I am not an expert at mold remediation. What I have written here, a lot of it, is just common sense. And, much of it is based on observing what the mold remediation company did in correcting the mold problem in my house. Some of it was learned through reading books on mold removal. Mold remediation is not rocket science and can be done on your own if you are careful and know something about construction or know enough to hire someone who knows. If you can afford it, a mold remediation company is the best way to go, to get the best results, safely. But I know that many people cannot afford a mold remediation company and might chose to either do it themselves with out any knowledge of what to do or opt to do nothing at all. Either case is bad and harmful to their health. So, by providing information on how to do mold remediation, yourself, but safely, I feel I am providing a needed service. Remember, this can be very dangerous without protection. A respirator is definitely a REQUIREMENT. A simple dust mask is not acceptable! On a recent episode of *Extreme Home Makeover*, they featured the family of five who lost their firefighter father to toxicity from exposure to stachybotrys while he had been renovating his moldy basement. He inhaled too many stachybotrys spores and it was fatal. Yes, in high enough amounts this stuff can kill you! So be CAREFUL!

Chapter 10
Summary

Toxic Black Mold Syndrome can be a very serious problem for many people. It seems that 25% of the population gets very sick, and remains so even upon leaving the mold contaminated building. But the rest of the population can get and remain sick if they remain in the mold-contaminated building. So it still can be a significant problem for everyone.

Buildings, both commercial and residential, can have toxic mold. And it isn't only old poorly maintained buildings that can have toxic mold. Newer construction can be just as bad! Many people in the market to buy houses only look at newer construction to avoid mold and don't realize that newer buildings might also have mold problems due to sloppy construction practices. New construction sometimes uses green wood that has moisture in it. Siding may be slapped up over wood that had been rained on and not allowed to dry. Insulation, left out in the rain, may be put into walls before being allowed to dry. Faulty plumbing or leaky roofs can lead to a steady supply of water to support mold growth. All these mistakes spell out mold disasters for the new homeowners. And these unlucky people won't even know what is making them sick. They will spend thousands of dollars seeing doctors trying to figure out what is wrong, while it is the house itself that is slowly sickening them.

There have been many reports of schools being contaminated with toxic molds. This is most likely due to poorly maintained school buildings because of inadequate funding for education. Reports of children affected by mold toxicity are disturbing.

I believe Toxic Black Mold Syndrome in this country is under recognized and is more common than most people believe. Most people have no idea that mold can make them sick. Some people are sick from toxic mold and do not know that mold is what is making them sick. It took me almost a whole year to figure out that toxic mold was making me sick! People need to be more aware of this problem and doctors and healthcare workers need to learn how to recognize the symptoms, diagnose it and treat it. The medical profession needs to recognize and admit that so many people, affected with similar symptoms, after exposure to toxic mold, cannot all be crazy. It is not just depression as doctors suggested to me. Neurological symptoms do not support the diagnosis of depression.

There is much research in animal studies showing the toxicity of mold mycotoxins. There, however, is limited clinical research on the human health effects of mold toxins. More research on the effects of toxic mold on humans is needed.

Laws need to be passed to protect citizens from the potentially devastating effects of toxic black mold. Right now, it's like the wild wild west, with toxic mold, the outlaw, being allowed to run rampant, while the sheriff just turns his back and ignores it. How many people must get sick? How much productive work must be lost? Toxic indoor mold needs to taken very seriously. It is just as dangerous if not more dangerous than asbestos. If left alone asbestos stays in one place. If toxic mold is left alone, it releases its spores, silently and invisibly, filling the air with its dangerous neurotoxins. How many lawsuits is it going to take? There is no doubt that indoor mold toxins are dangerous. Many have been found to be carcinogenic. Some may have been used or were considered for use in biological warfare! Doesn't any of this sound like a danger to human health.

Both the current stand by medical organizations that mold toxins are not proven to be a problem and the absence of any laws protecting citizens from toxic black mold, are causing many people who are the victims of toxic black mold poisoning to suffer even more than they already have. Not only are they struck with horrible symptoms, but they also have to cope with much financial loss, disbelief of their disease, and sometimes the loss of a job or a home.

References

Rosen, Gary, Ph.D. and Schaller, James, M.D. "Your Guide to Mold Toxins." Tampa, Florida Hope Academic Press, 2006.

Rosen, Gary, Ph.D. C.I.E. "Mold and Mold Toxin Remediation." Tampa, Florida Hope Academic Press. 2006.

Kaufman, Doug A. "The Fungus Link To: An Introduction to Fungal Disease Including the Initial Phase Diet." Rockwall, Texas: MediaTrition, 2000.

Kaufmann, Doug A. with Holland, David, M.D. and Clark, Jami, R.N. "The Fungus Link, Volume 2, Tracking the Cause." Rockwall, Texas: MediaTrition, 2003.

Kaufmann, Doug A. with Holland, David, M.D. and Clark, Jami, R.N. "The Fungus Link Volume 3 Know the Cause." Rockwall, Texas: MediaTrition, 2005.

Shoemaker, Ritchie C., M.D. with Schaller, James, M.D. and Schmidt, Patti, "Mold Warriors: Fighting America's Hidden Health Threat." Baltimore, Maryland: Gateway Press Inc. 2005.

Etzel, Ruth A. M.D., Ph.D., "Linking Evidence and Experience: Mycotoxins."

Johanning, Eckardt, M.D., M.S.C, "Fungal and Related Exposures." Occupational Medicine Secrets 1999.

Mumpton, Frederick A., "La Roca Magica: Uses of Natural Zeolites in Agriculture and Industry." Proc Natl Acad Sci USA 1999, March 30 96(7): 3463-3470.

Pavelic, K., et al., "Natural Zeolite Clinoptilolite: New Adjuvant in Anticancer Therapy." J. Mol. Med. 2001 78(12) 708-720.

Katic, M. et al. "A Clinoptilolite Effect on Cell Media and the Consequent effects on Tumor Cells in Vitro," Front Biosci 2006 May 1: 11 1722-1732.

Rodriguez-Fuentes, G., et al., "Enterex: Anti-Diarrheic Drug based on Purified Natural Clinoptilolite." Zeolites 19 441-448, 1997.

Kralj, M. and Pavelic, K. "Medicine on a Small Scale." EMBO Rep 2003 Nov 4(11); 1008-1012.

Martin-Kleiner, I. et al. "The Effect of the Zeolite, Clinoptilolite on Serum Chemistry and Hematopoesis in Mice" Food Chem Toxicol, 2001 Jul: 39(7) 717-727.

Ivkovic, S. et al. "Dietray Supplementation with the tribomechanically activated zeolite Clinoptilolite in immunodeficiency: Effects on the Immune System," Adv. Ther. 2004 March-April: 21(2):135-47.

Ambruster, Thomas, "Clinoptilolite-heulandite: Applications and Basic Research"

Shurson, G.C. et al. "Effects of Zeolite A or Clinoptilolite in diets of growing swine." J. Anim. Sci. 1984 Dec: 59(6):1536-45.

Pond, W.G., Yen, J.T., "Protection by clinoptilolite or zeolite NaA against cadmium-induced anemia in growing swine." Proc Soc Exp Biol Med 1983 Jul: 173(3):332-337.

Elmore, A.R. "Cosmetic Ingredient Review Expert Panel," Int J Toxicol 2003: 22 Supl 1:37-102.

Cousens, Gabriel, M.D., "The Natural Zeolite Product." Tree of Life Rejuvenation Center, Arizona Treeoflife.nu.

Voidani, A, et al. "Antibodies to molds and satratoxin in individuals exposed in water-damaged buildings." Archives of Environmental Health, July 2003.

Mercola, Joseph, M.D. "The Top -10 Myco-Toxic Foods," Mercola.com 2007.

Fungal Research Group Foundation, Inc. "Toxigenic stachybotyrs atra and other allergenic and toxic fungi," Fungalresearchgroup.com.

Johanning, Eckardt, M.D. et al. "Health and Immunology Study Following exposure to toxigenic fungi (stachybotyrs chartarum (atra) in a water damaged office environment." International Archive of Occupational and Environmental Health (1996) 68:207-218.

"T-2 Mycotoxins and Yellow rain: The same destructive neurological agent that is found in indoor molds," Mold-survivor.com.

Locasto, Donald A., M.D. "CBRNE T-2 Mycotoxins" Emedicine from webMD, emedicine.com.

Lillard-Roberts, Susan "Symptoms of Fungal Exposure (mycotoxicosis)," Mold-survivor.com.

Peraica, M, et al. "Diseases Caused by Molds in Humans; Bulletin of the World Health Organization," Sept 1, 1999, Healthandenergy.com.

Cummins, Joe, prof. "Increased Mycotoxins in Organic Produce?" Institute of Science in Society Press Release 11/23/04.

EHP online, "Mycotoxins: Of Molds and Maladies," January 14, 2004, healthandenergy.com.

Lillard-Roberts, Susan "Chaetomium," Sunday, Oct 3, 2004, mold-help.org.

"Ciguatera Fish Poisoning," Holistichealthtopics.com.

Armstrong, David "Amid Suits over Mold, Experts Wear Two Hats: Authors of Science Paper Often Cited by Defense, Also Help in Litigation," *The Wall Street Journal* Tuesday, January 9, 2007, Vol CCXLIX, No. 7 page A1 and A16.

WebMD.com, "Facts May Calm Mold Madness," Medical News Archive, Jan 26, 2007.

Brautbar, Nachman, MD, medical expert, practicing physician, university professor, "Toxic Molds Revisited (2006) Indoor Molds and their Symptoms," Environmentaldiseases.com.

"Anaphylaxis," mold-survivor.com

DeNoon, D. "Allergy Major Cause of 'Toxic Mold Syndrome,' But Many cases of mold-linked illness Not Allergy." WebMD Medical News, WebMD.com Feb 24, 2005.

Flappan, S.M., et al., "Infant pulmonary hemorrhage in a suburban home with water damage and mold (Stachybotyrs atra)." Environ Health Perspect, 1999, November; 107(11): 927-930.

Islam, Z., et al. "Satratoxin G from the Black Mold Stachybotyrs chartarum Evokes Olfactory Sensory Neuron Loss and Inflammation in the Murine Nose and Brain." Environ Health Perspect, 2006 July; 114(7): 1099-1107.

Christensen, C.M. et al. "Toxicity to Rats of Corn Invaded by Chaetomium globosum." Appl Microbiol. 1966 September; 14(5): 774-777.

Hayes, M.A. and Wobeser, G.A. "Subacute toxic effects of dietary T-2 toxin in young mallard ducks." Can J Comp Med. 1983 April; 47(2): 180-187.

Fan, T.S., et al. "Production and characterization of a monoclonal antibody cross-reactive with most group A trichothecenes." Appl Environ Microbiol. 1988 December; 54(12): 2959-2963.

Ezeonu, I.M., et al. "Effect of relative humidity on fungal colonization of fiberglass insulation." Appl Environ Microbiol. 1994 June; 60(6): 2149-2151.

Friend, S.C., et al. "Experimental T-2 toxicosis in sheep." Can J Comp Med. 1983 July; 47(3): 291-297.

Wakefield, Julie, "A Killer Smell: Mold Toxin Destroys Olfactory Cells in Mice." Environ Health Perspect 2006 July; 114(7): A428.

Harrach, B. et al. "Isolation of satratoxins from the bedding straw of a sheep flock with fatal stachybotryotoxicosis." Appl Environ Microbiol 1983 May; 45(5): 1419-1422.

Rao, C.Y., et al. "Reduction of Pulmonary Toxicity of Stachybotrys chartarum Spores by Methanol Extraction of Mycotoxins." Appl Environ Microbiol. 2000 July; 66(7): 2817-2821.

Yike, I., et al. "Mycotoxin Adducts on Human serum Albumin: Biomarkers of Exposure to Stachybotrys chartarum." Environ Health Perspect 2006 August; 114(8): 1221-1226.

Vesper, S.J., et al. "Quantification of Siderophore and Hemolysin from Stachtbotyrs chartarum Strains Including a Strain Isolated from the Lung of a Child with Pulmonary Hemorrhage and Hemosiderosis." Appl Environ Microbiol. 2000 June; 66(6): 2678-2681.

Mislivec, P.B., et al. "Mycological survey of selected health foods." Appl Environ Microbiol. 1979 March; 37(3): 567-571.

Jarvis, B.B., et al. "Study of Toxin Production by Isolates of Stachybotrys chartarum and Memnoniella echinata Isolated during a Study of Pulmonary Hemosiderosis in Infants." Appl Environ Microbiol. 1998 October; 64(10): 3620-3625.

Dearborn, D.G., et al. "Overview of investigations into pulmonary hemorrhage among infants in Cleveland, Ohio." Environ Health Perspect 1999 June; 107(Suppl 3): 495-499.

Sorenson, W.G. "Fungal spores: hazardous to health?" Environ Health Perspect. 1999 June; 107(Suppl 3)): 469-472.

Gravesen, S. et al. "Microfungal contamination of damp buildings—examples of risk constructions and risk materials." Environ Health Perspect 1999 June; 107(Suppl 3): 505-508.

Bata, A. et al. "Macrocyclic trichothecene toxins produced by Stachybotrys atra strains isolated in Middle Europe." Appl Environ Microbiol. 1985 March; 49(3): 678-681.

Vesper, S.J. and Vesper, M.J. "Stachylysin May Be a Cause of Hemorrhaging in Humans Exposed to Stachybotrys chartarum." Infect Immun. 2002 April; 70(4): 2065-2069.

Sorenson, W.G., et al. "Trichothecene mycotoxins in aerosolized conidia of Stachybotrys atra." Appl Environ Microbiol. 1987 June; 53(6): 1370-1375.

Kuhn, D.M. and Ghannoum, M.A. "Indoor Mold, Toxigenic Fungi, and Stachybotrys chartarum: Infectious Disease Perspective." Clin Microbiol Rev. 2003 January; 16(1): 144-172.

Murtoniemi, T. et al. "Effect of Plasterboard Composition on Stachybotrys chartaum Growth and Biological Activity of Spores." Appl Environ Microbiol. 2003 July 69(7): 3751-3757.

Brasel, T.L., et al. "Detection of tichothecene mycotoxins in sera from individuals exposed to Stachybotrys chartarum in indoor environments." Arch Environ health 2004 June; 59(6): 317-23.

Cooke, W.B. and Foter, M.J. "Fungi in Used Bedding Materials." Appl Microbiol. 1958 May; 6(3): 169-173.

Wakefield, Julie "National Meeting Breaks the Mold." Environ Health Perspect 2004 October; 112(14): A810-A811.

Vojdani, A. et al. "Saliva Secretory IgA Antibodies Against Molds and Mycotoxins in Patients Exposed to Toxigenic Fungi." Immunopharmacology and Immunotoxicology 2003 Vol 25, No.4: 595-614.

Fung, F. et al. "Stachybotrys, a mycotoxin-producing fungus of increasing toxicologic importance." J Toxicol Clin Toxicol 1998:36(1-2):79-86.

Fung,F. and Clark, RF. "Health effects of mycotoxins: a toxicological overview." J Toxicol Clin Toxicol. 2004; 42(2):217-234.

Gordon, KE. et al. "Tremorgenic encephalopathy: a role of mycotoxins in the production of CNS disease in humans?" Can J Neurol Sci 1993 Aug; 20(3):237-239.

Di Paolo, N. et al. "Acute renal failure from inhalation of mycotoxins." Nephron. 1993:64(4):621-5.

Creasia, DA., et al. "Acute inhalation toxicity of T-2 mycotoxin in mice." Fundam Appl Toxicol 1987 Feb; 8(2):230-5.

Brasel, TL. et al. "Detection of tricothecene mycotoxins in sera from individuals exposed to Stachybotrys chartarum in indoor environments." Arch Environ Health 2004 Jun; 59(6):317-23.

Hossain, MA. et al. "Attributes of Stachybotrys chartarum and its association with human disease." J Allergy Clin Immunol. 2004 Feb; 113(2):200-8.

Hodgson, MJ. et al. "Building-associated pulmonary disease from exposure to Stachybotrys chartarum and Aspergillus versicolor." J Occup environ Med. 1998 Mar; 40(3):241-9.

Johanning, E. et al. "Health and immunology study following exposure to toxigenic fungi (Stachybotrys chartarum) in a water-damaged office environment." Int Arch Occup Environ Health 1996; 68(4):207-18.

Leino, M. et al. "Intranasal exposure to a damp building mould Stachybotrys chartarum, induces lung inflammation in mice by satratoxin-independent mechanisms." Clin Exp Allergy 2003 Nov; 33(11):1603-10.

Yike, I. et al. "Acute inflammatory responses to Stachbotrys chartarum in the lungs of infant rats: time course and possible mechanisms." Toxicol Sci 2005 Apr; 84(2):408-17.

Dearborn, DG. et al. "Clinical profile of 30 infants with acute pulmonary hemorrhage in Cleveland." Pediatrics 2002; Sep; 110(3):627-37.

Etzel, RA. "Stachybotrys." Curr Opin Pediatr 2003 Feb; (1):103-6.

Etzel, RA, et al. "Acute pulmonary hemmorhage in infants associated with exposure to Stachybotrys atra and other fungi." Arch Pediatr Adolesc Med. 1998 Aug; 152(8):757-62.

Edmnson, DA. Et al. "Allergy and 'Toxic Mold Syndrome.'" Ann Allergy Asthma Immunol 2005 Feb; 94(2):234-9.

Khalili, B, et al. "Inhalational mold toxicity: fact or fiction? A clinical review of 50 cases." Ann Allergy Asthma Immunol 2005 Sep; 95(3):239-46.

Johanning, E., et al. "Health and Immunology Study Following Exposure to Toxigenic Fungi (Stachybotrys charatarum (atra) in a Water-Damaged Office Environment." Internat Arch of Occup and Environ Health 1996; 68:207-218.

McAnally, Tom. "Conference battles mold ailments." UMConnection Vol. 14, no.7, April 2, 2003.

Shoemaker, RC. "A Primer in Sick Building Syndrome: Lessons from the Somerset County District Court"

Shoemaker, RC. "Medical Problems...Arising from Environmental Conditions" Interview conducted by Wells Shoemaker BS, FAFS. Filtration News May/June, 2002.

Shoemaker, RC. "How Sick is your building...and what you can do about it?" Part 1. Filtration News May/June 2001

Shoemaker, RC. "Getting Behind 'Sick Building Syndrome.'" Filtration News July/August 2001.

Rogers, Sherry, M.D. "Detoxify or Die" Sand Key Company, Inc, 2002.

Dusseault,J et al. Evaluation of alginate purification methods:effect on polyphenol, endotoxin and protein contamination. J Biomed Mater Res A. 2006 Feb:76(2):243-51.

Wandrey,C. and Vidal, DS, Purification of polymeric biomaterials. Ann N Y Acad Sci 2001 Nov:944:187-98.

The Holy Bible, New King James Version 1994, Thomas Nelson, Inc.

Made in the USA
Coppell, TX
31 December 2019